Freeing Yourself from

Pelvic Pain

A Complete Self-Help Guide to Overcome
Pelvic Floor Disorders, Dyspareunia, Vulvodynia & other Symptoms

Claudia Amherd

The original edition was published in 2008 under the title "Wenn die Liebe schmerzt" by Books on Demand GmbH, Germany

1st edition
First edition in English (brit.): March 2013.

ISBN-13: 978-1505264050
ISBN-10: 1505264057

Translated from the German by tolingo GmbH
Picture/Ilustration credits: Claudia Amherd, E – Palma
Illustrations: Nadja Baltensweiler CH – Lucerne
Pictures: Herbert Zimmermann, CH – Lucerne
Cover Photo: detailblick - Fotolia.com

Note:
The contents of this book have been carefully examined and verified. However, the manual is not a substitute for a visit to the doctor! Neither the author nor her commissioner assume liability for personal injury, physical damage and financial loss.

For more info contact:
Claudia Amherd
Palma de Mallorca
Spain
www.moyosecrets.info

DEDICATION

For all the wonderful women, who have successfully beaten vaginismus thanks to their tremendous courage, openness and endurance. They and their open feedback have played a significant role in creating and developing the self-help and therapy programme "Vaginismus besiegen®" [beating vaginismus].

For all women, who pick up this book for the first time today and who have the courage to go on a journey of self-discovery that will lead to a life without vaginismus.

I wish you a good measure of curiosity, strength, endurance and many beautiful moments of sensual contact

CONTENTS

viii

PREFACE

When love hurts – do you know the feeling?

»I feel like my vagina has no opening at all.«

»My husband cannot penetrate. It's as if he were hitting a wall.«

»I'm scared of giving it another go. It simply doesn't work. I'm just in awful pain. I get this burning, stabbing sensation.«

»At my last gynaecological examination I cried like a little girl. It was so painful.«

These feelings are typical for women who suffer from vaginismus. Some women suffer for years without finding relief. Even professionals such as doctors and therapists are often only able to offer limited advice and support or none at all. Vaginismus is still an alien concept for many and a taboo issue in our society.

About three months after I started giving pelvic floor exercise classes, I was confronted with »dyspareunia« for the very first time. There was a woman, who was taking private pelvic floor exercise lessons with me. When I asked her for a letter of referral, she gave me a doctor's prescription. Diagnosis: dyspareunia. I had never heard of the term before, so my first move was to look it up in the medical dictionary. It read: »Dyspareunia: pain for the woman during sexual intercourse due to incompatibilty of the sexual partners.« This explanation did not really mean anything to me. I gave her gynaecologist a call, but that did not make the matter any clearer either. Back then, I was sadly unable to help this woman much. After a few training sessions she had to quit due to even greater pain.

This encounter somehow took hold of me, and thus my "research quest" through textbooks, studies, the internet, forums and congresses began. Later, I realised why this woman had complained about even greater pain. She suffered from extreme tension in her pelvic floor; through the training exercises, the already existing tension increased, which intensified the pain.

Thus began my journey to becoming an expert on treating women with vaginismus and similar conditions. Back then, as today, it was very hard to come by literature on vaginismus. Meanwhile, I gathered lots of experience in treating vaginismus. For more than eight years, I have been dealing with this topic on a daily basis. And time and again people ask me sheepishly: "Vaginismus? Never heard of it. What is it?"

With this book I would like to contribute to making the taboo topic of vaginismus public and socially acceptable. And above all, I would like to help women to beat vaginismus with my profound knowledge and with my therapy approach. It is high time that women stop thinking "There's something wrong with me" or "I am the only woman in the world who can't have sex, everyone else seems to manage".

This book is aimed at all these women. But I especially dedicate this book to all women and couples who have thus far trusted in me and who, thanks to their openness and courage, have helped to make my therapy "Vaginismus besiegen®" [beat vaginismus] what it is today: owing to these women and couples, it has become a knowledge-based, targeted and fully developed treatment with a great success rate. These women were able to celebrate many personal victories over vaginismus.

I hope that reading this book will also lead to your personal "beat vaginismus" success story.

With best regards, Claudia Amherd

HOW TO WORK WITH THIS BOOK

This book is an info book, a workbook and a self-help book with information, instructions and a complete self-help programme for women who suffer from vaginismus, dyspareunia or vulvodynia. This book is also for men, who would like to help their partner with overcoming vaginismus. But this book is also meant as an information and support book for psychotherapists, doctors and sex therapists who would like to offer their patients help and information around the topic of vaginismus.

PART 1 will inform, describe and explain causes, symptoms and treatment options for vaginismus, dyspareunia and vulvodynia.

PART 2 comprises a step-by-step guide through my treatment programme "Vaginismus besiegen®" [beat vaginismus]. You will reflect on your own "vaginismus story", train your pelvic floor, practise with vaginal dilators and get to know partner exercises. Work on one chapter at a time – because every single step is significant for your way to success and always builds on what you have learned in the previous chapter.

PART 3 answers questions frequently asked by women coming to my surgery.

PART 4 is aimed at professionals and people with an interest in medicine. The anatomical images are shown again with more detailed labelling. Further, you will get an overview of questions concerning changes in the diagnosis criteria for vaginismus, dyspareunia and vulvodynia that are currently being discussed among experts.

When you start with the exercises, first create a comfortable atmosphere in which you can practise in peace. Place everything you need within reaching-distance – that way you can work in a relaxed way and without interruption.

FREQUENTLY ASKED QUESTION

Q: **Can I really treat vaginismus on my own with this book?**

A: Yes! All exercises, instructions, information and aids you need to "treat yourself" can be found in this book. Thanks to the many responses I got from women who have successfully overcome vaginismus with this book, I can safely say: it works!

The benefit of this book, and consequently your success, depends on how many of the exercises you put into practice or can put into practice. It is quite possible that, because you spent years searching for a term that describes your affliction or for a treatment option, you are somewhat anxious, and you may need some time before you feel you can begin with the training. You may need courage to embark on this journey to yourself, to your own body and to your own sensuality. You may need to be brave to conquer yourself, to follow your own intuition and to listen to your body and the signals it sends out. Or maybe you will need support – be it from your partner, your best friend or from an experienced therapist. Take all the time and space you need. Allow yourself to fulfil your personal needs, and make sure you get all the support you require to progress and to succeed.

"I had already been practising with the dilators for two years. But I never knew that pelvic floor exercises help to make the routines with the dilators painless. Now I can at last also practise with the third and fourth dilator."

"After my doctor gave me a prescription for the Amielle-Set, I tried to practise with the dilators. But it was always very painful. After a while, I practised less and less frequently and finally, disappointedly, I abandoned the dilators. I thought I would never make it. But with the instructions and the many tips for vaginal training I was at last able to successfully practise with the dilators."

"For the last eight months, I have worked with your book and have well and truly beaten vaginismus. Now I thoroughly enjoy having sex with my husband and am two months pregnant!"

Q: **How long will it take for me to overcome vaginismus?**

A: That varies a lot from woman to woman. My intensive programme "Vaginismus besiegen®" [beat vaginismus] can completely beat vaginismus in 14 or 21 days. Women who have a weekly appointment with me or with a genito-pelvic pain therapist trained by me, or who want to overcome vaginismus with the help of this book, usually take three to twelve months. Frequent difficulties are day-to-day life as well as strain related to the job, the social environment and the family. Practising 4-5 times a week and facing up to vaginismus requires a lot of strength. Emotionally, mentally, psychologically, but also physically. When you begin with the self-help programme, be sure to go at your own pace; stay motivated and be very patient with yourself. Your progress depends on various factors. For example: how regularly do you find time to practise? Do you have a partner who supports you, or do you practise on your own? Do you suffer from other physical or psychological conditions such as irritable bowel syndrome, fears or depression? How committed are you to your job?

Q: Can I also work with this book if I suffer from dyspareunia or vulvodynia?

A: Yes. If you suffer from vulvodynia, it may be sensible to also use other aids, as described in the chapter on vulvodynia. To achieve permanent pain relief, you will need a little more patience and endurance than women who treat vaginismus. You can also beat dyspareunia with this self-help programme. Pay your doctor a visit to rule out or to treat conditions such as endometriosis or an infection of the vagina.

Q: I am single. Can I beat vaginismus all the same?

A: Yes, of course! As a single woman, you can still practise steps 1 to 6 of my treatment on your own. In the course of the programme you will for example learn to use tampons, and you will be able to go to a gynaecological examination. And you will gain certainty. And certainty will give you confidence in your own body, which will in turn prepare you for a future relationship.

PART 1
INFORMATION
ON DYSPAREUNIA,
VAGINISMUS AND
VULVODYNIA

Contents

Research into vaginismus and vulvodynia is sadly still in its infancy. Information is hard to come by, and treatment options or studies are difficult to find. Women suffering from the condition often try to get a diagnosis or treatment for years – because even experienced gynaecologists sometimes fail to make the diagnosis. The information gathered here shows: you are not alone. You are not the only woman, who suffers from this condition. And you are not abnormal. Your body simply reacts differently from other women's bodies. And with patience and practice, you will become one of the women who have successfully beaten vaginismus.

DYSPAREUNIA

Dyspareunia is the medical term for pain during sexual intercourse. Any sort of pain that occurs while making love can be summed up with this word. Vaginismus and vulvodynia are specific forms of dyspareunia, but cannot always be clearly defined as something separate. The pain may occur upon penetration, during and/or after sexual intercourse. The pain can affect all parts of the genital area. The labia, the vagina, the clitoris, the vulva, the perineum. The sensation may be a burning, stabbing, searing, itching, or it may come in spasms. Equally varied is the location of the pain during sexual intercourse. The woman may feel it deep inside, in the outer third of the vagina or upon penetration.

Note: there is currently a lively discussion among professionals about how to define and properly classify dyspareunia, vaginismus and vulvodynia in the next edition of the DSM-V [1] . The definitions and descriptions presented in this book comply with the current guidelines regarding diagnosis and classification of the standard works DSM-TV-TR (2000) and ICD-10 (2007).

What is the difference between vaginismus and dyspareunia?

Diagnostically, it is often impossible to distinguish between vaginismus and dyspareunia. In practice, vaginismus is seen as a special form of dyspareunia, but sadly this diagnosis is still not made often enough. In the case of vaginismus, the pelvic floor muscles tense up, which causes the vagina to narrow, resulting in pain when trying to insert a finger, tampon or speculum. Penile-vaginal penetration is painful or simply

---

1 Diagnostic and Statistical Manual of Mental Disorders published by the American Psychiatric Association. 2 International Statistical Classification of Diseases and Related Health Problems published by the World Health Organisation (WHO).

impossible. In the case of dyspareunia, it is not the tensing up of the pelvic floor muscles that causes the pain. Instead, there is another physical reason *(organic dyspareunia)*. If the cause of the pain is unknown or if the pain persists although an inflammation of the vulva, vagina or uterus has long since gone down, the condition is called *non-organic dyspareunia*.

However, in the case of dyspareunia, the pelvic floor can still be affected. The pelvic floor muscles often tense up when pain occurs due to inflammations or other disorders around the genital area. These cramps sometimes persist, although the original disorder has long since passed. This condition is called *secondary vaginismus*.

POSSIBLE CAUSES FOR DYSPAREUNIA

There are countless possible causes for dyspareunia. It is not uncommon that the couple's sexual practices are the cause for pain during sexual intercourse: there may be too little arousal due to non-existent or too short foreplay, due to lack of tenderness, listlessness or positions in which the man penetrates too deeply.

Vaginismus, vulvodynia or dyspareunia can occur together with other disorders around the genital area. However, once the cause, the basic problem, has been eliminated, pain during sexual intercourse may still persist. These symptoms then require a careful treatment.

Frequent causes for dyspareunia are:

- Too little time spent on foreplay, too little sexual arousal (dryness of the vagina)
- Inflammation of the urethra and the bladder
- Vaginal inflammations (e.g. Gardnerella), vaginal thrush
- Dry vagina
- Interstitial cystitis (bladder pain), injuries from giving birth
- Scar tissue in the genital area
- Falling of the womb
- Gynaecological operation
- Radiotherapy in the area of the pelvis, the thighs, the abdomen
- Genital tumours, cysts
- Endometriosis (endometrial material in other tissues), salpingitis, cysts of the Fallopian tubes
- Painful gynaecological/urogynaecological examinations
- Allergic reactions (condoms, body wash, clothing, spermicides etc.)
- Cysts of the Bartholin glands
- Vulvodynia
- Vulvar vestibulitis
- Vaginismus

THIS IS HOW DYSPAREUNIA CAN BE TREATED

The treatment of dyspareunia is as varied as its causes. First of all, it is important to find out exactly why the woman is suffering from pain. If infections, falling of the womb, tumours or other disorders can be ruled out, the same treatment as for vaginismus is the sensible way forward. So, if you suffer from dyspareunia, you can follow the self-help programme with pelvic floor exercises, relaxation, vaginal training and partner exercises step by step exactly as described in this book.

Following operations, radiotherapy or severe injuries, it is best to do the dilator training with the Amielle Care set. For a list and contact details of retailers, see the appendix. If you are unsure which set is the right one for you, don't be shy to call Owen Mumford or the P6 Beckenboden-zentrum [pelvic floor centre] for more information.

VAGINISMUS

What is vaginismus?

In the case of vaginismus, the vagina is extremely touch-sensitive. A woman suffering from this condition experiences real difficulties when inserting a finger, tampon or penis, although she wishes to do so. When trying to insert something, the muscles around her vagina (pelvic floor) tense up involuntarily. This tension arises automatically. The woman does not do this on purpose. The tension of her pelvic floor muscles can sometimes be so strong that inserting her own finger or a tampon or having sexual intercourse becomes impossible.

Pain or a burning or stabbing sensation accompany any attempt at inserting something. The pain, however, is only temporary or situation-related. As soon as the woman stops trying to insert something, the pain subsides. Many women suffering from these cramps of the pelvic floor do not feel their pelvic floor muscles contract. Instead, they feel as if their vagina was closed or as if they had no opening at all.

There are many forms of vaginismus. Some women are fine with having a gynaecological examination but cannot have sexual intercourse. Other women are neither able to have a gynaecological examination nor to have sexual intercourse nor to insert a tampon.

Medically speaking, vaginismus is currently classed as a sexual pain disorder. Vaginismus is not a venereal disease, it is not infectious, it is not a mental illness and it cannot be sexually transmitted. The genitalia are completely normal and in working order! Nor is the vagina too small. The vagina is very, very stretchy. After all, a baby can squeeze its way through the vagina during birth.

And the good news is: vaginismus is highly treatable. The global numbers and my own success rate of well over 90 per cent speak for themselves.

DIFFERENT TYPES OF VAGINISMUS

Vaginismus can affect younger or more mature women, women with years of sexual experience or women with no sexual experience. If a woman already has difficulties during puberty with inserting a tampon or having a gynaecological examination, she suffers from primary vaginismus. If she complains about pain during sexual intercourse after an operation or after she has given birth, she suffers from secondary vaginismus.

Degrees of severity of vaginismus

Not all women suffer from the same symptoms. The symptoms of vaginismus come in different forms which are categorised into four degrees of severity:

I Vaginal penetration and thrusts of the penis give the woman discomfort. She feels a burning sensation and tightness. The pain, however, subsides during sexual intercourse.

II A stronger burning sensation with tightness upon vaginal penetration. The discomfort persists.

III The unconscious contraction of the pelvic floor muscles makes vaginal penetration and penis movement difficult and painful.

IV The pelvic floor muscles contract so severely that the opening of the vagina is closed. If penetration is forced, the woman experiences gruelling pain.

Primary vaginismus means that a woman already suffers from vaginismus during her first ever attempt at having sexual intercourse. Typically, the woman realises that she has "problems", i.e. vaginismus, when she first tries to have sex. It is impossible for the man to enter into the vagina. He feels "as if he were hitting a brick wall", where normally the opening of the vagina should be.

Many women also have difficulties inserting a tampon or having a gynaecological examination. Also other medical procedures or examinations in the genital area can prove to be very difficult: for example an examination of the urethra, inserting a catheter into the urethra or anal examinations.

What women affected by primary vaginismus frequently say:

"The examination was very painful. The doctor really hurt me. I cried with pain. I never want to have a gynaecological examination ever again."

"I've never been able to have proper sexual intercourse. It's always been so painful. Something is definitely wrong with me."

"The doctor said I'm fine. So why do I have this awful pain?"

Secondary vaginismus usually occurs later in life, after a longer period of "pain- and problem-free" sex. In most cases, vaginismus follows on directly from painful disorders in the pelvic and genital area. A woman can enjoy years of pain-free sex. But then, after a vaginal infection, the pain persists. Even after the treatment has been completed and the infection has passed, the pain remains. The woman then suffers from pain during sexual intercourse and displays typical symptoms of vaginismus. For some women the condition can become so severe that they can no longer insert a tampon or undergo a gynaecological examination.

Typical triggers for secondary vaginismus are:

- A difficult birth, injuries to the perineum
- Operations in the genital area, vaginal operations
- Radiotherapy of the genital area, the pelvis or the thighs
- Infections, such as recurring urinary tract infections, inflammation of the vagina
- Endometriosis (endometrial material in other tissues)
- Vulvodynia
- Exposure to violence
- Sexual abuse, rape

What women affected by secondary vaginismus frequently say:

"When he starts to move, it is so painful that he has to stop."

"Since the birth of our child it just doesn't work anymore. When he tries to enter, I become so tight that I get these gruelling, stabbing pains."

SYMPTOMS OF VAGINISMUS

Depending on the degree of severity, the symptoms of vaginismus range from a burning sensation during sex to the impossibility of inserting anything into the vagina. The following list will give you an overview of possible symptoms. Some women suffer from one or two of these symptoms, other women suffer from several of these symptoms at once.

- You are unable to insert you finger, or you feel pain when inserting your finger.

- You have difficulties or experience pain when inserting a tampon.

- Vaginal penetration is difficult or impossible.

- Penile-vaginal penetration is painful or very uncomfortable.

- You avoid sexual intercourse, because it is very painful or impossible.

- You experience a burning or stabbing sensation, a dragging pain or tightness during sexual intercourse.

- You have suffered from enduring pain during sexual intercourse since having given birth, since having had an operation such as hysterectomy (removal of the uterus), cancer operations or operations to beat incontinence etc.,

since having had urinary tract infections, vaginitis/vaginal thrush.

- You have not yet had sexual intercourse although you are married or are living with a partner.

- Gynaecological examinations are very painful for you or even impossible. You suffer from pain, tension or cramps in various groups of muscles, for example in your legs, shoulders, back, neck, lower back and pelvis.

- Since you experienced psychic and/or physical trauma – such as physical or sexual abuse, violence, rape – you suffer from ongoing pain or difficulties during sexual intercourse.

Do I suffer from vaginismus?

Q: I don't feel any pain when my partner penetrates me. But once he starts moving, I get this burning sensation, and it gets worse and worse until I have to stop because it is just too painful. Do I really have vaginismus?

A: Yes. If your gynaecologist does not detect any other physical cause, you can assume that you suffer from a moderate form of vaginismus.

Q: I get this feeling of tightness when having sex. But it subsides after a while. Is that vaginismus?

A: Yes. This is a mild form of vaginismus. So you can still benefit from the exercises. They will help you eliminate the feeling of tightness upon penetration.

8

Q: Having sexual intercourse hurts. Especially if he penetrates deeply. But I don't get this feeling of tightness.

A: No. This is dyspareunia. Make an appointment with your gynaecologist to look into possible causes for your pain.

Q: I suffer from permanent pain. Sometimes I can hardly work.

A: No. This is vulvodynia.

Accompanying symptoms of vaginismus

- Many women are afflicted with irritable bowel syndrome, constipation and/or haemorrhoids.
- Frequently recurring urinary tract infections (inflammation of the urethra, inflammation of the bladder) either in your youth/adolescence or also currently.
- Frequently recurring infections of the female genitalia, e.g. vaginal yeast infection, vaginal inflammations.
- Painful bowel movement and/or painful anal examinations.
- Pain when having an examination of the urethra or when a catheter is being inserted.
- Menstrual pain.
- Fears, stress, nervousness, severe tension.
- Problems with the jaw area, grinding of teeth.
- Muscle cramps in areas other than the pelvic floor.

THESE REASONS MAY LEAD TO VAGINISMUS

There are many reasons why a woman may be suffering from vaginismus. Quite often, there are several reasons at once. Some reasons are physical, others are mental or psychological. But it is not uncommon that no reason for the condition can be found. To successfully treat vaginismus, it is unimportant whether you have actually found your personal reason or not. However, understanding vaginismus and unearthing possible causes for it may help you to accept and overcome the situation.

Be it physical, mental or without cause – vaginismus occurs unconsciously. A vicious circle of pain, fear and muscle response that tightens the vagina. Often, a woman's body reacts with vaginismus due to a combination of mental and physical causes:

when trying to have sex, the body expects pain. The body, especially the pelvic floor, wants to shield itself against the pain and tenses up. The vagina tightens. Consequently, it becomes even more painful, when the man tries to penetrate – the body tenses up even further ...

Pain induces fear. Once this cycle has started, fear of pain develops. Already the thought of inserting something raises fears. Fear is not "only" a feeling. Like with all feelings, the body also reacts to fear. The muscles, especially the pelvic floor, tense up, you may break into a sweat, get diarrhoea, a stomachache ...

Mental/psychological causes that may trigger vaginismus:

- **Fear of becoming pregnant.** The fear of becoming pregnant is quite common in young women, who know very little about sexuality and contraception. Often, these young women hear about how a cousin, friend or sister got pregnant by accident. They are then pressurised by parents etc.: "Don't you dare get pregnant, too."

- **Fears relating to the hymen.** Young women are often consumed by the fear that the hymen will have to be painfully pierced when they experience their "first time". Sometimes the fear of an agonising tearing and heavy bleeding during her first sexual intercourse is so strong that the woman's whole body, and especially her pelvic floor, tenses up so completely that her vagina closes and her partner is unable to penetrate.

- **Fear of surrendering control.** Many women who suffer from vaginismus are deeply committed to their job and their social environment. They organise their work and private life to a T. Sexuality not only entails the tenderest form of communication with yourself or with your partner, but also implies partly relinquishing control over your body and mind. Arousal and orgasm are impossible without relaxation, without devotion and without surrendering control over your own body somewhat.

- **Stress, emotional stress,** feelings of guilt because of sexuality, unhealthy or negative attitude towards sexuality, lack of sex education, negative sexual experiences in the past. Stress can trigger many physical reactions. It is important to find a positive way of dealing with stress. A negative approach towards tenderness and sexuality in general can also cause pain during sex. The body simply no longer wants to have these "negative" experiences.

- **Problems in the partnership**, fear of becoming dependent on the partner, fear of surrendering control, mistrust or lack of faith. Women with vaginismus are often afraid of devotion. Or they are afraid of becoming dependent on their partner. Most women are also afraid of losing control or doing something "bad".

- **Trauma, emotional consequences of rape, physical and psychological violence,** suppressed experiences. Physical consequences are one aspect of violence, but mental and emotional reactions are also possible.

- **Childhood experiences, lack of sex education,** strict religious upbringing ("sex is bad"), confrontation with pornographic images, inadequate sex education. Too strict an upbringing in which sexuality is not discussed in an adequate and child-friendly way can cause a lot of damage. A positive self-image, also in relation to a girl's sexuality, can thus be nipped in the bud. But the opposite is also true: a girl can become worried if she is confronted with sexuality too early. Some women recount experiences that overwhelmed them as a child. For example, they saw pornographic material without knowing what was coming. Or they found their parents' sex toys without realising that their parents were hav

- **Pregnancy and birth, a difficult birth,** injuries from giving birth (episiotomy), delivery with the help of forceps or a ventouse, caesarean section. Giving birth can seem very traumatic for a woman. The muscle memory registers:something is brutally penetrating my vagina (= pain). The body does not want to experience this trauma again and "closes up". Some doctors make a negative remark about the woman during delivery or while stitching the episiotomy. For example, when the woman failed to have an enema beforehand and is a little soiled. Or

when she has not yet been cleaned up after having given birth. This behaviour can seriously stress the woman, even if she does not consciously take in these remarks.

- **Illnesses, medical causes** such as urinary tract infections, falling of the womb, falling of the bladder, tumours or cysts on the genitalia, vulvodynia, vulvar vestibulitis, infections of the uterus or the vagina etc. Such disorders can involve considerable pain. Here again, the body wants to protect itself against more pain and reacts accordingly. Vaginismus continues, even if these disorders have long since passed.

- **Pelvic operations,** accidents and injuries in the pelvic area, difficult or painful gynaecological examinations. Operations, accidents and injuries can have a traumatic effect on the body. Sometimes we do not realise how much an operation/injury really hurt us mentally. Painful examinations at the gynaecologist can trigger vaginismus or worsen an existing condition. This of course also inclu-des other examinations around the woman's genital area. For example, examinations of the urethra (placing a catheter) or anal examinations.

- **Medication.** Some drugs are known to cause muscle cramps or pain as side effects.

- **Physical abuse,** physical or psychological violence, rape, sexual/physical/psychological abuse, beating. Traumatic experiences can trigger vaginismus. For example, sexual violence, but also other physical and/or psychological violence. It does not always have to be sexual abuse. Other experiences of violence can also trigger vaginismus.

Even though the above list includes experiences of violence, sexual abuse and rape as possible causes for vaginismus, not every woman suffering from the condition has necessarily lived through one of these traumatic experiences. In other words, not every woman with vaginismus has experienced sexual or other violence. Studies show that the number of women who suffer from vaginismus is no greater among victims of sexual violence than among other women. After all, every third woman experiences sexual violence or sexual assaults at some point in her life.

Possibly, you will find other (or additional) causes that have led to your personal case of vaginismus.

HOW COMMON IS VAGINISMUS?

There are only very few studies that deal with vaginismus. Some surveys that deal with sexual disorders in general also provide numbers on dyspareunia and vaginismus. Depending on the study, dyspareunia apparently affects 3 to 43 per cent of all women. It is thought that 1 to 8 per cent of women suffer from vaginismus, although the estimated

number of undetected cases is almost certainly significantly higher. By way of comparison: 6 per cent of the world's entire population suffers from incontinency (bladder weakness), most of them women.

Looking at these numbers, it becomes clear how many women and couples are suffering from vaginismus, some of them for years. You are not the only woman/the only couple fighting vaginismus. And: vaginismus is definitely beatable.

THE HYMEN

Are there women who have difficulties with sexual intercourse due to their hymen?

Very, very, very rarely. Difficulties with sex due to the hymen is much, much less common than difficulties due to vaginismus! Every woman is different, and so is every hymen. However, the defloration horror stories with heavy bleeding are, in most cases, fairy tales.

What is the hymen?

The hymen is a layer of tissue at the entrance to the vagina. This delicate layer of tissue partly closes the vagina. So the hymen is not actually located inside the vagina, but on the outside and belongs to the external genitalia.

A female foetus's vagina is initially completely closed with this thin layer of tissue. Shortly before the baby girl is born, however, this tissue divides and becomes the hymen.

Every girl's hymen is different in size and form. Many hymens cover the entrance to the vagina in a ring-shape. Other hymens are perforated, like a strainer. Some girls no longer have a hymen when they are born, because the tissue has already completely divided.

In over 50 per cent of young women, the hymen has already (often unnoticed!) been torn before they engage in sexual intercourse for the first time. If it is stretched little by little over a longer period of time, for example through the use of tampons or masturbation, the hymen may become so elastic that a penis can penetrate without rupturing it. Many women still have remains of the hymen until their first child is born.

Q: **If the hymen is indeed so stretchable and delicate, where do the stories about defloration come from?**

A: The concept of defloration has its origin in a time in which young women were actually still girls when they were married off. Often, they were forced to marry men, who were quite a few years older. And that a grown man injures a girl, when he penetrates her, is obvious. A girl, whose body is still developing, has much more tender genitals. Such injuries can be very painful and may bleed.

A girl may bleed a little on her »first time«, but not necessarily. Often, the "first time" is full of new, unknown and unfamiliar emotions. Some women may also find it a little painful. Especially, if both partners are inexperienced. But generally, this feeling of pain will go away with more experience.

Imperforate hymens

Very, very rarely, it happens that a woman's hymen has hardly any opening or is indeed completely closed. If a young woman does not seem to get her period at all, this may hint at an imperforate hymen, i.e. a hymen without an opening. In this case, the woman may have similar symptoms to a woman suffering from vaginismus. Here, a surgical opening of the hymen may be necessary. This is a simple procedure, a very fine cut, which is carried out under anaesthetisation. Once the cut has healed, the woman will be free of symptoms.

THIS IS HOW VAGINISMUS CAN BE TREATED

Pelvic floor exercise

The tightness in the vagina is caused by tensed up pelvic floor muscles. Women, who suffer from vaginismus, have a constantly increased base tension in their pelvic floor without sensing that they are tensing their muscles at all. Generally, they lack a conscious awareness of their pelvic floor muscles. Thus they cannot tense or relax their pelvic floor of their own volition. Once a woman starts training her pelvic floor correctly and specifically, the base tension goes down and she can consciously tense and relax her pelvic floor.

Not all forms of pelvic floor exercise are suitable for treating vaginismus. Many classes teach how to create the kind of tension that leads to vaginismus or that worsens the symptoms of vaginismus. The pain will get worse, and there will be no beneficial effect at all.

You will learn how to train your pelvic floor correctly in Step 2, in the practical section of this book.

Biofeedback

With biofeedback, electrodes are stuck on your pelvic floor. This will help you to learn to relax your pelvic floor. You will be able to see on a screen, whether you are tensing or relaxing your pelvic floor and how strongly you are tensing your muscles. Once you are able to insert something into your vagina, you can insert a probe. Here, once again, the intensity with which you are tensing your pelvic floor will be displayed on a screen.

Biofeedback will really help you learn, whether your pelvic floor is tensed or relaxed.

Vaginal training

Traditionally, vaginismus is treated with vaginal trainers (dilators). Here,

women train their vagina to get used to the sensation of penetration. The aim of training does not consist of stretching the vagina, but to regain control over the opening of the vagina.

Initially, you insert small dilators into your vagina. Then, gradually, you go over to using larger and larger ones, until you reach the size of a penis. Using lots of lubricant is a must, as this facilitates inserting the dilators.

The vaginal training should not cause any pain, but a light burning sensation may occur. Some women try to train their vagina with dilators, dildos or other objects without any sort of guidance. As they keep feeling pain, they continue to train their body memory to think "penetration equals pain". Therefore, do not use the vaginal trainers before you have learnt the techniques with which to relax your pelvic floor. Otherwise, you will only unnecessarily worsen your condition.

In Part 2 of this book, in the manual for self-treating vaginismus, you will find detailed instructions on how to practise with the dilators.

Psychotherapy

Psychotherapy probably seems like a sensible addition. But psychotherapy alone cannot treat vaginismus. Because vaginismus is not a mental illness. Many women visit their psychotherapist for years, and yet the symptoms of their condition remain.

Some professionals are convinced that vaginismus is psychosomatic, i.e. that vaginismus develops due to a psychological defence reaction. And in some cases, this in undoubtedly true. There is definitely a psychological component to vaginismus. However, the "main part" of vaginismus is physical. That is why it makes sense to treat vaginismus in a physical way. Ideally, vaginismus is treated holistically. In other words, a treatment programme should equally take into account relationship patterns, psychological components and the physical part.

So, seeing a psychotherapist while battling vaginismus may indeed be a sensible move for some women. But dyspareunia, vaginismus or vulvodynia cannot be cured by psychotherapy alone.

Sex therapy

Vaginismus is not really a classic sexual disorder, but a pain disorder. Sex therapy can help a woman to re-evaluate and redefine her attitude towards sexuality. Some women who suffer from vaginismus have a negative attitude towards sex or very little sexual experience. In these cases, a sex therapy can help to clarify things or help to resolve negative thought patterns. Here, the woman can learn new patterns of behaviour. Couples may want to go to a sex therapist together. This will help them to be more open about their sexuality, teach them to communicate with trust and to attend to one another's needs and wishes.

Sex therapy can encourage a woman to explore her own body with pleasure, especially after a successful vaginismus therapy. For most couples, just a few therapy sessions are enough to get them back on track for a future of sensual and enjoyable sex.

However, these measures alone will not cure vaginismus. They lack the physical aspect, the work on body perception and the targeted training of the pelvic floor.

Botulinum toxin

Botox® is a neurotoxin that is produced by bacteria. In recent years, there have been a few attempts at treating vaginismus and vulvodynia with botulinum toxin. The success rate is very high, however, the only study on this topic to date is rather small (25 women took part, 24 were successfully treated, Iran 2004).

With this treatment, Botox® is injected into the woman's pelvic floor, i.e. directly into the tensed up muscles. The muscles are then paralysed for 2 to 4 months. During this time, the woman can engage in vaginal training with dilators and get used to having painless sex. The muscle memory relearns. Once the effect of the Botox® injection wears off, the vaginismus should be overcome. To completely beat vaginismus, you may need repeated injections. However, doctors explicitly state that Botox® should only be used if all other possibilities have been exhausted.

How does vaginismus affect your partner?

Vaginismus and the resulting sexual difficulties can put a huge strain on all levels of a relationship. If you work through the vaginismus programme as a couple, this experience may greatly enrich your relationship and strengthen your partnership. Although it is the woman who is suffering physically and mentally under vaginismus and its painful consequences, the partner usually suffers in almost equal measure. In addition, it often takes weeks, months or even years before vaginismus is diagnosed and a satisfactory solution can be found. The strain on the partner is immense. He often feels just as desperate, helpless and frustrated as the woman. In many partnerships, all attention is focussed on the woman's condition, and the man's needs are neglected or blocked out. Some men are unable to bring up the courage to voice their feelings and thoughts for fear of hurting their partner. But to find a solution to the condition, it is also incredibly important to talk about unpleasant feelings the partner may have, because feelings can make up part of the problem, too.

The following statements by men do not all make for pleasant reading. Some might even frighten you. Nonetheless: you will need to come to grips with this aspect. Perhaps you should read and discuss the quotes and advice together with your partner. But please do not start pointing blame!

Instead, be thankful to one another for being so open. Remember: you are standing at the beginning of a new era. The two of you will have to live through a few hard weeks, but at the end you will have gained so much, both individually and as a couple.

Partners of women with vaginismus often describe their feelings as follows:

Feelings of guilt

Many men feel guilty towards their partner. Some men are under the impression that it is their fault that their partner suffers from pain or that they are unable to have sex. Some men also feel guilty just for wanting sex.

"I feel bad, because I still want to have sex with her, even though I can see how much she suffers."

Many men cannot bear to see their partner suffer, when they are trying to have sex. Nonetheless they would love to be intimate with their partner.

"I love her. So, is it selfish to want sex with her?"

Frustration

"I'm really making every effort to understand her. But what about me? I have feelings, too."

Many men would love to have sex and enjoy the intimacy, trust and satisfaction that sexuality can bring. Sex can forge a connection, can bring reconciliation and can make up the tenderest, most intimate form of communication between two people. Sexual activity also distinguishes a love relationship from a deep friendship. It is frustrating to have to deny oneself all the advantages that sexuality has to offer.

Pity, empathy

"My wife would die of shame if anyone knew about 'her' vaginismus. I'm so sorry for her, because she is in such pain. I know she loves me and that she doesn't want to hurt me. But her problem is hurting us both. I don't know what to do."

Anger

"Okay. I'm not always the supportive and understanding partner I should be. Sometimes I'm mad at the vaginismus, mad at my partner, mad at couples who can have normal sex. Sometimes I'm just generally mad at everything. It's driving me insane, when she rejects me and doesn't want my affection. When I remember that it isn't really her fault, I stop being mad at her – but deep down inside, I am somehow still furious."

At some point, many couples completely stop being intimate. They concentrate on the problem of penetration not working and are sadly no longer able to enjoy other forms of intimacy.

Rejection

"I no longer want to be rejected all the time. What's wrong with me? Why doesn't she want me in a sexual way? At first, sex just wasn't possible. But now I get the feeling that she no longer wants sex. I think she finds me unattractive."

Detachment

"My private life is a complete mess. I sometimes don't even want to see my wife at all. I am happiest when I can bury myself in my work or when I can spend time with my friends. When I'm away or busy I don't always have to think about it."

Fears

"I don't know for how much longer I can stand this. I love my wife, but honestly: I don't want to spend my whole life in a partnership without sex. Besides, we wanted children. But if we don't sleep together, how is that ever going to happen? I don't know where this vaginismus will lead us and what our future holds."

It is important that your partner understands what vaginismus is. That he gets to know the emotional and physical background. He should also know that vaginismus can be beaten and that you have started a programme that will help you to do so. Take as many steps as possible together with your partner. This will give your partner a task and will enable him to actively help solve the problems. If you take the steps of the programme together, you will both find it a lot easier to reach the final step.

VULVODYNIA

Literally translated, vulvodynia means "pain of the vulva", i.e. of the woman's external genitalia. Women who suffer from vulvodynia generally also feel pain during sexual intercourse. Vulvodynia mostly affects younger women between 20 and 40 years of age. A typical sign of vulvodynia is a constant pain of the labia or the perineum. This pain also makes cycling, sports or sitting difficult. Vaginal penetration, inserting a tampon or sexual intercourse are usually impossible.

DIFFERENT TYPES OF VULVODYNIA

Several disorders fall under the umbrella term of vulvodynia. In practice, however, they are rarely distinguished and are often used synonymously. Examples are vestibulitis, vulvar vestibulitis or vestibulodynia. In recent years, the diagnoses has been made more frequently, especially when women suffer from pain around their genital area with no known cause.

Vulvodynia in younger women

(vestibulodynia/vulvar vestibulitis)

The woman suffers from pain, a burning or stabbing sensation or acute irritation of the vulval vestibule (vestibule of the external genitalia). Your doctor will diagnose you with vulvodynia if the following factors apply:

Lightly touching the vulval vestibule causes a burning or stabbing sensation or pain.

Light pressure with a cotton bud triggers the symptoms.

The vulva is more or less reddened between the five and seven o'clock position.

The symptoms have been persistent for more than 6 months. Just like with vaginismus, the term *primary vulvodynia* is used for when the symptoms appear when the woman first becomes sexually active (10 to 20 per cent of women who suffer from this condition). The term *secondary vulvodynia* is used for when the symptoms only develop after a longer symptom-free period.

Vulvodynia in women aged 40 and over

(vulval dysaesthesia / general vulvodynia).

In most cases, women suffer from dysaesthesia shortly before, during or after menopause. Women with this condition report a burning sensation or pain. The symptoms are chronic and crop up spontaneously without plausible cause. The condition affects the whole vulva; often also the urethra or the rectum. Women with urinary and faecal incontinence frequently show symptoms of vulvodynia.

THE ROLE OF THE PELVIC FLOOR IN THE CASE OF VULVODYNIA

If a woman has vulvodynia, her pelvic floor is weakened, which leads to tension in the muscles. When starting with pelvic floor exercises, these muscles lack endurance, and the difference between tension and relaxation is very small. That is to say tension and relaxation lie close together – the woman can neither properly tense nor relax her pelvic floor.

THIS IS HOW VULVODYNIA CAN BE TREATED

The self-help programme for vaginismus is also effective in combating vulvodynia. You will need a lot of patience to overcome vulvodynia, because a therapy takes at least six months, and for the pain to go away completely, it often takes even longer. If you suffer from enduring or very strong discomfort, you may need an additional drug-based treatment.

Ideally, your doctor and therapist will cooperate and try to find solutions together with you.

Pelvic floor exercise

Pelvic floor exercise is also an important part of treating vulvodynia. Usually, the pelvic floor is very weak and tensed up. It is important to start very gently with the pelvic floor exercises, so as not to increase the pain.

Relaxation

Simple relaxation techniques not only reduce muscle tension but also help manage stress and pain. Learn a relaxation technique that suits you and practise it daily. In the practical part of this book, you will learn progressive muscle relaxation, PMR for short. This is a very easy relaxation technique that can be practised daily without a huge amount of time.

Vaginal training

Relaxing the pelvic floor, which can be achieved with vaginal training, reduces pain permanently and effectively. The greatest difficulty is often the fear of pain and injury.

Medication

Antidepressants: in today's pain management, a low dose of tricyclic antidepressants is often used as a painkiller. The drug is taken over a limited period of time – in the case of vulvodynia, a treatment usually takes four to six months. You start off with a very low dose. The dose is increased every week, until an effective pain reduction kicks in.

Soothing ointments: lidocaine 5 % is used to great success. The cream is best applied generously, covered with gauze or cotton wool and left alone over night. It is recommended that the cream is left on the affected area for at least eight hours. For a significant pain reduction, lidocaine should be used daily for at least 8 weeks.

Biofeedback

Pelvic floor exercise with the help of a gadget: electrodes are attached to the perineum, or a vaginal probe is inserted into the vagina. You then tense and relax your pelvic floor muscles and the device will show you how strongly you are tensing/relaxing your pelvic floor muscles. An experienced therapist can help you by putting together training programmes that are suitable for combating vulvodynia.

Operations

It is not uncommon that women with vulvodynia are advised to undergo surgery. In this case, the affected skin area is removed. But as the pain points often migrate, the operation does not always bring the desired relief.

MORE HELPFUL TIPS FOR WOMEN WITH VULVODYNIA

- Avoid synthetic underwear. Choose cotton underwear instead (even though the designs are not always very sexy).

- Coloured underwear is often treated with irritating substances.

- Wear loosely fitting underwear. Thongs can irritate the area additionally.

- Use unbleached and undyed toilet paper.

- Soap and douches, deodorants, wet wipes etc. contain irritating substances and throw the vaginal flora out of balance. Wash the external genital area with a ph-adjusted soap or with a special intimate wash. Wash the interior of the vagina with water only.

- Take a shower rather than a bath.

- Do not wash several times a day.

- Personal hygiene of the genital area is best undertaken without flannels or brushes.

- When doing your laundry, dispense with fabric softeners and other additives. Possibly rinse underwear twice.

- Avoid sports that increase the pain, e.g. horseback riding or cycling.

- Change out of your wet bikini/bathing costume immediately after swimming.

- Some women find coldness soothing. Carefully wrap up some ice and gently apply to the painful area for a few minutes.

HINTS FOR USING THE SELF-HELP PROGRAMME AGAINST VULVODYNIA

You can work through the whole self-help programme step by step, because it is ideal for combating vulvodynia. You will need a lot more patience and endurance, and in some instances you may need additional aids such as prescription drugs or special ointments. But your success will make up for it. Keep a pain diary during your training. See below for how this works:

The pain diary

	Monday	Tuesday	Wednesday	...
	4/10	4/11	4/12	...
Morning	Pain 2	Pain 2	Pain 1	
Note	after getting up	after getting up	after getting up	
Midday	Pain 5	Pain 5	Pain 4	
Note		a day off, after a stroll trough town with a friend	during conference	
Evening	Pain 3	Pain 2	Pain 3	
Note		after pilates	applied ice	

Scale of pain

0   No pain
1   Light burning sensation, hardly noticeable
2   Stronger burning sensation or light pain, also perceivable without focussing on the pain point
3   Persistent, but bearable burning sensation or feeling of pain
4   Moderate pain, with effect on your overall condition
5   Stronger pain, annoying, sitting is uncomfortable
6   Stronger pain, even a light touch is painful
7   Intense pain, day-to-day activities are only partially possible
8   Very intense pain, hardly bearable, working and/or concentrating is only partially possible
9   Agonising pain, great despair
10 Unbearable pain, accompanied by aggression and depression

You can also make notes in your pain diary about what forms of pain relief you tried – to see what worsened your condition and what worked. On the one hand, the pain diary will help you judge the degree of pain you are experiencing, on the other hand, it will also show you the progress and success of the treatment. Keep a pain diary for a week so that you get an overview of your perception of pain. This way, you can also give your doctor or therapist a guide to your pain and to how it progresses.

Also keep your pain diary, when you start with the self-help programme and make a note of your pain, for example, before and after the pelvic floor training, the relaxation exercises or the vaginal training. When doing your pelvic floor and vaginal training, please make sure you don't exceed the pain threshold of 3 (pain diary!).

TIPS FOR DOING YOUR PELVIC FLOOR EXERCISES

As, in the case of vulvodynia, your pelvic floor muscles are not only weakened and tensed up, but as they also lack endurance, be sure to begin especially gently with the pelvic floor exercises. Start with only one exercise and carry it out slowly and accurately. When you feel you are tensing up, stop the exercise, pause for a moment and relax, then begin again.

The juggling ball hurts

If the juggling ball induces stronger pain than that described in category 3 – a persistent, but bearable burning sensation or feeling of pain – then leave out the juggling ball to begin with. Instead, do a contact exercise standing up:

- Stand with your feet hip-width apart. Hip joints and knees are vertical to one another.

- Bend your knees. Take care that your knees remain behind your big toes.

- Lean your upper body forward, keep it ramrod straight.

- Take one or both hands and feel for your sitting bones. The sitting bones are located roughly in the centre of the natal cleft, exactly where the bottom merges into the thigh, somewhat to the middle towards the perineum.

- Contract the sitting bones towards the perineum. You will be able to feel with your fingers how the muscles between the sitting bones and the perineum tense and slightly contract towards the perineum. Relax, contract sitting bones towards perineum, relax, contract sitting bones towards perineum (pulsate).

- Pulsate as often as you like. If possible, start off with five to ten pulsations. Do not be afraid to just pulsate three to five times in one go. At the beginning of the training programme, most women suffering from vulvodynia are unable to do more pulsations without increasing their pain or without tensing up. So, when treating vulvodynia, always keep in mind: less and short is more! Relax for a moment and then repeat the contact exercise again.

- A variation of the exercise: scrutinise the movement of your pelvic floor with a hand mirror when pulsating. The perineum should contract very slightly and arch inwards a tiny bit. Continue with these two exercises, until you feel your pelvic floor. You can practise for three minutes today, for five minutes tomorrow and for ten minutes the day after tomorrow. Your body determines how often, for how long and how intensively you can train your pelvic floor. It is better to train only a little to begin with and to then slowly increase your programme. After a while, you will know exactly how best to structure your training sessions.

Intensity of the pelvic floor training

To ensure the training does not worsen your pain, please take care to exercise very cautiously and thoroughly to begin with. But above all: exercise with minimum force and be really gentle!

Only do about five to ten pulsations (tense and relax pelvic floor) at first, take a short break, then repeat. If you can do this without any problems, increase the number of pulsations.

If you feel you are tensing up, break off the exercise and start again from the beginning.

The contact exercises from the section "Discovering and waking up the pelvic floor" should be carried out in short units at first: two to five minutes are quite enough to begin with. Then slowly increase your exercise time until you can easily keep going for fifteen minutes.

Train with ease, precision and as softly as a feather, and you will increase the effectiveness of the exercises.

Vaginal training

The combination of pelvic floor and vaginal training is the most efficient form of pain relief for vulvodynia, provided you respect your personal pain threshold and do not overexert yourself. The fear of pain is often even greater in women suffering from vulvodynia than in those suffering from vaginismus. The vicious circle is already well established: fear of pain provokes stress. The pulse quickens, breathing becomes constrained, the muscles – not only the pelvic floor muscles – tense up. Therefore, it is important that you carry out the training extremely carefully; the exercises suggested under the heading of "Mental training" will be a real help with overcoming your fear.

Under no circumstances should the dilator training increase the pain. If you are unsure, please refer to the scale of pain (see page #21). Ascertain your level of pain according to the scale before training. Determine the level of pain again during and after the vaginal training.

Relaxation, pelvic floor training and inserting your own finger are a must before beginning vaginal training with dilators.

Try out the different forms of vaginal training and choose the one that suits you best. For example, choose a form of vaginal training in which you leave the dilator inserted for a long time. Move the dilator gently from time to time. Usually, the burning sensation/the pain is less severe if you always move the dilator very carefully.

It may be a good idea to apply ice on the painful area before a training session. Please wrap the ice in a soft cloth so as not to damage the skin around your genital area.

If pain-free exercising with the vaginal trainers is absolutely impossible, apply some relaxing lubricant or a soothing ointment, such as lidocaine cream 5 % (only available on prescription) around the entrance to your vagina.

Once you are already somewhat practised in vaginal training, you can use the training exercises as effective pain relief on days when you are in especially severe pain. Usually, gentle pelvic floor exercises in combination with vaginal training are more effective against pain than painkillers or pain-numbing ointments. So, don't be afraid to use the vaginal training to soothe your pain!

If you feel worse after training, you may be exercising for too long, too intensively or with too large a dilator.

Simply give several methods a go to see what is most helpful for you personally. However, do not keep changing from one method to another. Follow one strategy for several consecutive days to make sure you do not irritate your genital area more than necessary and worsen your condition.

PART 2
SELF-HELP PROGRAMME:
BEAT VAGINISMUS IN 7 STEPS

My seven-step treatment programme "Vaginismus besiegen®" [beat vaginismus] is based on four main pillars:

❖ Understanding Vaginismus

❖ Pelvic Floor Training

❖ Relaxation

❖ Partner Exercises

Contents

UNDERSTANDING VAGINISMUS

Here you will learn what vaginismus is and how the condition may come about. Take a look into your past: your own, personal history may help you overcome vaginismus. If you recall the past, you can make out your very own, personal experiences that have led to your case of vaginismus. You can assemble your personal treatment programme.

PELVIC FLOOR TRAINING

The pelvic floor plays a central role in treating vaginismus. Its base tension and its tasks are closely connected to the optimal function and health of the internal and external genitalia.

RELAXATION

In the case of vaginismus, not only the base tension of the pelvic floor is raised. Often, the body's entire muscular system is tensed up. For most women, fear is a constant companion. Relaxation will also help you to deal more calmly with fears.

PARTNER EXERCISES

At the beginning of the treatment, you will practise on your own. If you have a partner, tackle the last part together with him. Step by step, you will learn "the transition" from practicing with the dilators to enjoyable sex.

The following treatment programme will lead you through the entire treatment in 7 steps. You will be gently guided and accompanied through all steps. Should you need more support, you will find a list of therapists who have been trained by us under www.genito-pelvic-pain.com.

I wish you every possible success on your journey to yourself and to an open and sensuous sexuality without pain.

STEP 1:

UNDERSTANDING VAGINISMUS

This is what you will learn in the first step:

❖ You will understand what happens in the event of a vaginistic reaction.

❖ You will get to know the muscle memory.

❖ You will look back on your own, personal past in relation to vaginismus.

❖ You will discover possible causes that may have led to your case of vaginismus.

Contents

WHAT HAPPENS WHEN I SUFFER FROM VAGINISMUS?

If you suffer from vaginismus, your body is terrified of penetration. For some reason, your body has learned to be afraid of penetration, because it is painful. Every time you try to insert something, your body signalises: watch out, here comes pain! The muscles around your vagina – the pelvic floor – contract. They effectively want to save you from the pain. As a rule, other parts of your body are also affected and tensed up. Especially your bottom, the inside of your thighs, your stomach, shoulders, jaw, diaphragm and feet. Many women also hold their breath.

These body reactions take place unconsciously, like blinking, when an insect flies into your eye. But instead of saving you from pain, the tension causes the burning, stabbing, searing sensation – in other words pain – to increase all the more. Sometimes, the muscles contract so strongly that your partner cannot penetrate at all and that inserting a tampon or even your own finger becomes impossible. Although the vaginistic reaction should really save you from pain, it does the complete opposite.

Vaginismus is not down to a disease or a deformity of the female genitalia. Nor is the vagina too small or too narrow. Even though some women or doctors may sometimes get this impression. In many cases, the woman's pelvic floor tension constricts the vagina so much that the entrance to the vagina becomes invisible.

THE MUSCLE MEMORY

Many of our sequences of movement are in fact types of "learned reflexes". These are complex movements that are made up of many individual movements. Our brain would be completely overtaxed if it had to control every one of these tiny movements individually.

An example: when, as a child, we learn how to write, everything happens very consciously. First of all we learn how to draw lines, circles and hoops. Then, our hands and fingers learn highly complex movements –

they learn how to form the individual letters. And then they learn how to write words. At first, a child still needs to concentrate hard, when learning to write a new word. But after a while, we think of a word and simply write it down. Even when we encounter new words, we no longer think about how, for instance, the letter A is written. Perhaps, we think about which letters we must write, but then we just start writing. Another example is walking. A child still has to learn slowly and laboriously how to put one foot in front of the other. It needs to keep balance and keep an eye on the direction. Our body makes countless smaller and bigger movements, all of them running in the right order. If we had to consciously control every muscle and every movement when walking, our brain would be unable to cope. That is why our body uses something that could be called "learned reflexes". So, when we want to get from A to B, our bodies starts to move in a perfectly coordinated manner.

Muscle memory and sexuality

This may surprise you, but some of these "learned reflexes" also happen during sex. The manner of a touch, a special scent, a fantasy – these are sensory perceptions that trigger certain emotions within you and your body. Ideally, you feel pleasure. At worst, you feel disgust and tension. Over time, due to experience and conversations, every couple develops its own individual form of body communication. The partners learn what they like, what feels good and how they can give one another sensual pleasure. Muscles and the nervous system appreciate these feelings and emotions. Over time, the body switches to autopilot: a certain impulse is automatically followed by certain reactions.

While making love, your body takes in countless emotions and stimuli that are processed by your nervous system with the help of previous experiences

and your feedback. Normally, sexual experiences become more and more pleasurable and enjoyable over time. Your body relaxes, enables your partner to penetrate and experiences sexuality / sexual intercourse as sensual and arousing. Not only real experiences, but also images, fantasies and imaginings – both positive and negative – influence the way you feel about having sex and are very powerful. Sometimes so much so that adverse "learned reflexes" develop.

The fear of a painful "first time" can be so dominant that the body, and especially the pelvic floor, tenses up completely, every time you try to insert something. It may also be the case that a woman has undergone a painful gynaecological examination. The body then links this "experience" with every form of inserting something into the vagina.

WHY DO I SUFFER FROM VAGINISMUS?

The causes for vaginismus are as varied as the women who suffer from it. In most cases, it is impossible to discern "the" cause. Instead, there are several physical, emotional or mental factors that trigger the condition.

In order to treat vaginismus successfully, it is not important to find out the exact causes. Most women, who have successfully beaten vaginismus, are unable to make out a precise cause. My experience also shows that digging too deep in a woman's past can hinder rather than further the treatment. Negative experiences, injuries inflicted by partners, doctors and therapists and frustration about the sometimes many years of fruitless searching for explanations can overwhelm a woman so much that she has difficulties allowing new and positive thoughts and body experiences.

However, a short review of the own sexual history, on negative body experiences, on blocking thought patterns etc. can help you to accept your own situation and recognise, if vaguely, possible causes for vaginismus. Many women are relieved, when they realise that they are neither an unusual nor mentally ill person nor that they need to have experienced a suppressed incident of abuse to suffer from vaginismus.

WRITE DOWN YOUR PERSONAL HISTORY

Collect your sexual experiences, body experiences, relationship experiences and thoughts in a personal diary. These records should be exclusively for you. Not for your partner, not for your doctor, not for your therapist. That way, you can be truly open and honest with yourself, without shame or fear of humiliation.

■ What was the climate like at home with regard to intimacy, sexuality and the body?

■ How did you experience your parents in terms of intimacy and affection?

■ Did you ever have a bad experience during medical examinations or treatments?

■ Have you ever had difficulties with your bladder or bowel, pelvis or jaw (for example grinding of teeth)?

■ What were your past romantic relationships like in terms of intimacy, affection and sexuality?

■ Are you a total perfectionist? Do you dread making mistakes?

■ Do you dislike giving up control? Are you afraid of losing control?

■ Do you dread becoming pregnant or giving birth?

■ Do you sometimes suffer from panic attacks?

■ Have you had humiliating or violent experiences?

■ What are your thoughts on intimacy, sexuality and partnership?

Do not dwell on these questions for too long and do not search too far afield. Above all, write down things that are at the forefront of your mind, things that seem important to you. This way, you will get a clear picture that will help you to recognise possible personal reasons for why you suffer from vaginismus.

The "Tagebuch Vaginismus besiegen®" [beating vaginismus diary] offers additional help with writing down your history. Here you will find additional questions and guidelines, and you can write down your thoughts immediately. The diary is available separately or as part of the training kit "Vaginismus besiegen®" [beat vaginismus].

Note: should this review cause difficulties or should you reach your limits with regard to your emotions, support from a psychologist or sex therapist may help.

FOR YOUR NOTES

STEP 2:

DISCOVERING THE PELVIC FLOOR

This is what you will learn in the second step:

❖ Why the pelvic floor plays such

❖ an important role in treating vaginismus.

❖ What and where the pelvic floor is.

❖ How to tense and relax the pelvic floor purposefully and in a controlled manner.

❖ Which pelvic floor exercises will help you to relax your pelvic floor.

Contents

The pelvic floor and vaginismus are inextricably linked. The pelvic floor is a group of several muscles that work together. The vagina also lies embedded in the pelvic floor. If the vagina closes, when you try to insert something, this is down to the pelvic floor muscles, which tense up. The vagina becomes tight; you feel a burning sensation or pain. Get to know your pelvic floor muscles. Observe the difference between tension and relaxation. Gradually reclaim control over your love muscles. This ability will break the vicious circle of "penetration = tension = pain = fear = more tension".

Jenny, 37, Lucerne

"At the very beginning of the intensive programme, I was introduced to the contact exercise with the juggling ball. The exercise was painful and I was hardly able to sit (I couldn't even bare two seconds on the juggling ball). Claudia then gave me a thin mat to sit on. She told me to place my index and middle fingers under my sitting bones and to consciously push them together and to actively contract them the same time. That already felt a lot better. Then, as I went home, I had my eureka moment. I was finally able to feel how I could tense and relax my pelvic floor. My daily task for the following week was to think as often as possible about my pelvic floor and to sense whether it was tensed or relaxed. After a few days, I had my next eureka moment: regardless of whether I was crossing the street, cooking my dinner of sitting in my office chair, my pelvic floor was always tensed. And I also suddenly remembered something about my childhood. As a little girl, I hardly ever went to the toilet. I wanted to play and didn't want to risk missing anything. And right up to the treatment programme, I still only went for a wee 1-2 times a day, although I drink two to three litres of water every day. Claudia explained to me that the pelvic floor is tensed when holding back urine and that people usually go to the toilet 4-8 times a day. Today, I am convinced that this constant tension was one of the causes for my condition. The pelvic floor training has helped me a lot with managing the dilator exercises and to consequently beat my vaginismus."

WHAT IS THE PELVIC FLOOR?

The pelvic floor is an ingenious network of muscles in your crotch. It spans between the pubic bone, the coccyx/the sacrum and the sitting bones. At the front, it is connected to the stomach via the pyramidalis (a small muscle above the pubic bone), to the back it is connected via the coccyx and sacrum, and in the pelvis it is connected to the legs via the hip muscles around the hip joints. The pelvic floor participates in almost every movement of your body – only the delicate hand muscles are practically independent.

The tasks of the pelvic floor are manifold:

The pelvic floor muscles give you control over your bladder and bowel and save you from conditions such as falling of the bladder, bowel and womb. They enable you to insert your finger or tampons, to have gynaecological examinations and to enjoy sexual intercourse. They help you with giving birth and they allow you to have orgasms.

The pelvic floor is very flexible. It is always alert and a little tensed, so as to be able to react quickly and fulfil its tasks. This permanent light tension is called muscle tone. In women with vaginismus and vulvodynia, this muscle tone is constantly raised. The nerves that trigger the tension or relaxation in the pelvic floor react to many impulses from the body, the mind and from emotions. Based on experiences and previously learned reactions, the nerves decide how the pelvic floor acts and reacts.

An example: you feel the urge to urinate and need to go to the toilet. The bladder passes on this information to the pelvic floor: "I am full and I would like to relieve myself." To urinate, the pelvic floor needs to relax. At the same time, the pelvic floor receives this message from the brain: "I can't see a suitable place to urinate yet, the bladder will have to wait." The nerves order the pelvic floor to stay tensed so that the bladder remains shut. Once you have found a toilet, you can urinate. The pelvic floor relaxes. Now assume you are unexpectedly interrupted. Your pelvic floor muscles immediately tense again to stop you urinating – until you are once more undisturbed.

As a child, you probably experienced the following: you were desperate to go to the toilet, but you were unable to hold it in until the right moment. Despite making an immense effort, you could not prevent the little accident. Something similar happens in the case of vaginismus. You would like to insert your finger or a tampon. But the pelvic floor muscles react unconsciously with tension and do not allow relaxation.

In this step you will learn to consciously control your pelvic floor again. You will be able to distinguish between tension and relaxation and you will learn how to induce one or the other deliberately. Your muscles will learn new reaction patterns and relax, when *you* want them to.

AN ALL-ROUNDER IN THREE LAYERS

Your pelvic floor is as large as both your hands put side by side and as thick as your palm:

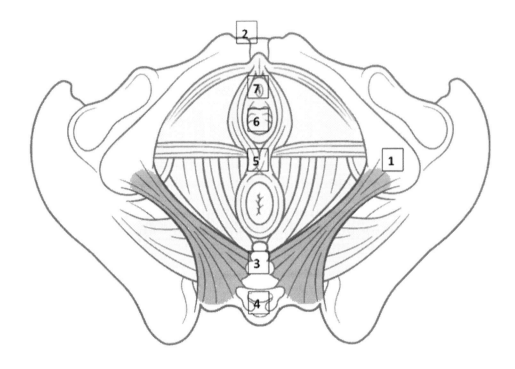

1 sitting bone
2 pubic bone
3 coccyx
4 sacral bone

5 perineum
6 opening for the vagina
7 opening for the urethra

THE OUTER OR LOWER LAYER

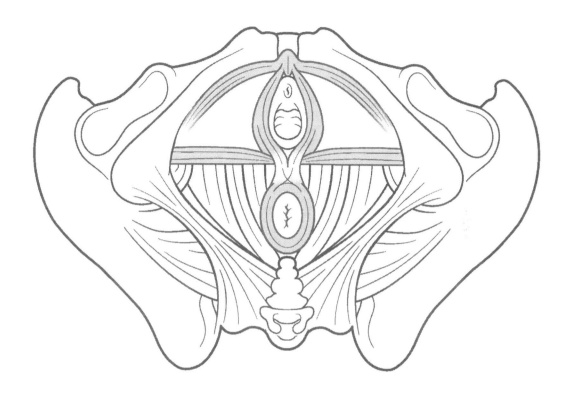

➡ more details page #123

The outer layer of the pelvic floor is the tenderest. This layer should not be explicitly trained, as it is extremely soft and delicate. If it is over-trained (which sadly happens with most forms of pelvic floor exercise), your vaginismus and pain during sex will worsen. This outer layer of the pelvic floor runs in a figure of eight from the pubic bone to the coccyx. Its delicate muscles run under the outer labia and over the Bartholin glands. The frontal loop encompasses the vagina and the urethra, the hind loop the anus. In the perineum, the frontal and hind loop cross. In addition to the figure-of-eight loop, there are two delicate muscles that run from the sitting bones to the clitoris and cover the crura ("legs") of the clitoris. If this layer is tender and supple, it increases arousal when stimulating the clitoris, encourages vaginal lubrication and causes the clitoris and labia to swell.'

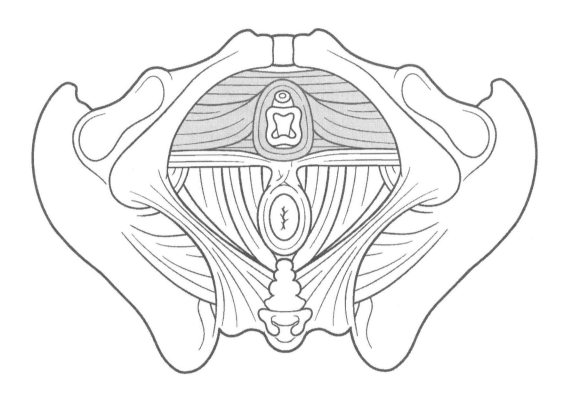

➠ more details page #124

The middle layer of the pelvic floor runs across from sitting bone to sitting bone. It closes the entire frontal area between the perineum and the pubic bone in form of a triangle. The urethra and vagina are embedded vertically into this layer of muscles. The middle layer is considerably stronger than the outer layer. And it plays a sgnificant role in causing the vaginistic reaction of the vagina. The middle layer is responsible for continence and prevents a falling of the bladder or womb. It is connected with the inner and outer layer in the perineum. When engaging in vaginal training, women often perceive this layer as a type of "sphincter".

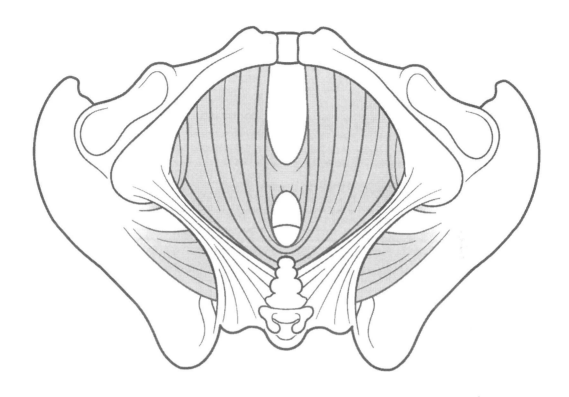

➡ more details page #125

The inner layer of the pelvic floor is the strongest and largest layer of all. It is connected to the coccyx at the rear, to the pubic bone at the front and to the sitting bones at the sides. It has the shape of a little basket. In the event of a "vaginal orgasm", the inner layer pulsates. The inner layer is often weak and severely tensed up. This causes pain deep down inside the vagina. The middle and inner layer of the pelvic floor affect most sex-related sensations and play a key part in sealing the vagina in the case of vaginismus.

DISCOVER AND WAKE UP YOUR PELVIC FLOOR

What do I need for training? A chair with a flat, hard seat – ideally a stool – and a juggling ball.

What type of juggling ball should I use? To prevent pain, the juggling ball for the contact exercise should not be too big. We usually use two sizes: a smaller ball to start off with, and a larger ball for when the tension in the pelvic floor has already gone down significantly. The ideal size for the small ball is a diameter of 4.5 cm (1.8 in), the larger ball should have a diameter of about 5.5 cm (2.2 in). It may be useful to know that this type of ball is frequently called "bean bag", should you want to buy yours in a specialised juggling shop. The size is often stated in grams, not in centimetres (inches). The smaller juggling balls generally run under the name of junior bags and weigh approx. 60g, the larger juggling balls tend to weigh 110g or 130g. Of course you can also order your juggling balls from the online shop on our homepage.

The benefits

- The awareness for the pelvic floor is raised.

- The pelvic floor is strengthened and becomes more reactive, the high degree of constant tension is lowered.

- The middle and inner layer of the pelvic floor are activated.

- Get away from the "tube feeling" – the "enemy" of vaginismus.

- Relaxing the pelvic floor will enable you to engage in painless dilator training.

- As the pelvic floor is part of a network of muscles connecting the pelvis, stomach, back and legs, the exercises will also relax your other muscles.

- Get up close and personal with your pelvic floor, gradually make friends with your genital area.

THE BASE EXERCISE: THIS IS HOW IT WORKS

1 **Take off your shoes** and sit down on – yes, you are reading correctly – the juggling ball. You are sitting exactly right, if you are touching the juggling ball with your perineum. The perineum is the area between your vagina and your anus. Sit with a good posture and in a relaxed way: your feet are under your knees, your knees hip-width apart.

2 **Direct your attention to your feet.** Gently push the balls of the big toes and the outer edge of your heels into the ground. Release. And again, push the base joints of the big toes and the heels into the ground. Really softly, really gently. The toes remain relaxed. Relax your knees, relax the inside of your thighs, relax the front of your thighs. Repeat this exercise until you feel a gentle pull, a twitch in the area of your sitting bones.

3 **Repeat once again:** push the outer edge of your heels and the balls of your big toes gently into the ground, until you feel a tiny pull that runs from the rear of your legs to the sitting bones. Relax your knees, relax the front of your thighs. Toes remain relaxed. Then hold this gentle tension.

This is how it should feel:

- Around the perineum, between the sitting bones, you feel a slight tension.

- Your bottom cheeks are relaxed and soft. When you place your hands on your bottom while you contract the sitting bones, your bottom remains soft and unmoving.

- The inside of your thighs and your groin are relaxed.

- Your breathing is calm, your stomach is soft and relaxed.

No-gos – this is what you should avoid:

- Tube feeling: you contract your labia and pull them inwardly/upwardly You feel tension in your vagina. Your vagina feels tight.

- You feel a slight burning sensation in the perineum or in the vagina. You hold your breath and cannot

4 **Veeeery, very gently, contract the sitting bones** towards the perineum, towards the juggling ball.

Release, contract, release, contract, release. 30 times, 40 times, 50 times ... Ever so gently, contract your sitting bones so that you can only just sense that you are moving something at all.

This is what you can do:

- Be even more gentle when contracting the sitting bones. Be really kind to yourself, to your body.

- Do not be ambitious. The more "sluggishly" you contract your sitting bones, the better!

ACTIVATE YOUR ENTIRE "PELVIC FLOOR BASKET"

The benefits

- You train your entire pelvic floor, which is interconnected with the stomach, back and pelvis.

- Tensions are balanced out: a weak pelvic floor is strengthened, tensions are slowly resolved.

- Your circulation is activated, internal and external genitalia are supported in their function.

- You can consciously tense and relax your pelvic floor – the most important thing for overcoming vaginismus!

THE "PELVIC FLOOR BASKET": THIS IS HOW IT WORKS

1 **Start in the same way as before.** Sit upright, place your feet exactly under your knees, knees hip-width apart. Gently push your feet – balls of your big toes and heels – into the ground, toes and knees remain relaxed. Feel the gentle pull along the rear of your legs towards the sitting bones. Take up the tension around the sitting bones.

2 **Move your sitting bones backwards,** move your pelvis/lower back to go into a slight hollow back position.

3 **Very softly, contract your sitting bones.** Gently hold the tension in your pelvic floor. Immediately go out of the hollow back position. Gently pull your coccyx and pubic bone vertically towards the floor – as if a weight were pulling down your coccyx and pubic bone.

4 **Connect your pelvic floor with your stomach:** establish tension in your perineum and pull ultra-gently towards the pubic bone. The pull should run past the urethra and the vagina on both sides, without tensing up the vagina or inducing the "tube feeling". If you do not succeed straight away: picture the exercise in your headnd repeat this a few times. You will see that your body will follow your thoughts, without any further assistance.

5 **Connect your pelvic floor with your back:** establish tension in your perineum and, as lightly as possible, pull backwards past the anus and towards the coccyx, relax the anus. If you have difficulties imagining this, take another look at the images of the layers of the pelvic floor to refresh your memory.

6 **Relax your back lengthwise,** vertebra by vertebra. A little more every time you exhale. Grow a few centimetres.

7 **Relax your shoulders** and shoulder blades and, gently, with hardly any effort, drop them outwardly and downwardly. Extend your neck, keep your chin at a right angle to your neck.

8 **Pulsate:** gently contract your pelvic floor muscles star-like from all sides towards the perineum. Release slightly, but do not release the tension completely. Contract again immediately, release slightly, contract, release slightly. 20 times, 30 times, 40 times. At the end, consciously release the whole tension.

What is the tube feeling?

The tube feeling sets in, when you press your labia together and pull the muscles around your vagina sharply inwardly. Or imagine interrupting the urinary stream when having a wee. Your bottom tenses, and your vagina feels cramped, like a tube. You hold your breath, your upper abdomen feels hard. You are welcome to give this a try so that you can properly appreciate the difference to the exercises above.

STARTING YOUR TRAINING SESSIONS

What you have learned so far, are the absolute basics, so-called contact exercises. I call these exercises "activating the pelvic floor". These "basics" make up the elementary foundation for the following pelvic floor exercises, in which you will activate and train your pelvic floor in various positions. Practice the following variations for a few days, until you can consciously tense and relax your pelvic floor. Until you are able to interlink your pelvic floor with your stomach and back. Only proceed to the next exercises, when you are sure you have "found" your pelvic floor! By all means, rely on your intuition. If your body feels light, relaxed, warm and comfortable, you are in the right place. This way, you will be able to do the following exercises with ease.

VARYING THE BASE EXERCISE: THIS IS HOW IT WORKS

Sit down on your juggling ball. Activate your pelvic floor basket as described before: softly contract your sitting bones. Link the tension towards the front with the pubic bone, towards the back with the coccyx, interlink the pelvic floor with the stomach and the back. With hardly any strength at all, stretch your back vertebra by vertebra. Slightly open your mouth, relax your forehead. Carefully move your shoul-

ders outwards and lower them backwards and downwards.

Pulsate with the rhythm of your heart

1 **Activate your pelvic floor,** connect the tension of the perineum with the pubic bone at the front and with the coccyx at the back. Stretch your spine, gently move your shoulders to the sides and lower them backwards and downwards.

2 **Pulsate with the rhythm of your heart:** very gently, increase the tension star-like from all sides towards the perineum, release slightly, increase tension, release slightly.

3 *Repeat 30 times.* After a few days, increase to 100, 200, 300, 400 pulsations.

Pulsate in slow motion

1 **Activate the pelvic floor:** sitting bones towards the perineum.Link the perineum towards the front with the pubic bone, towards the back with the coccyx.

2 **In slow motion,** slightly release the tension in the pelvic floor, then, very slowly, increase the tension again, then slowly release again.

3 **30 pulsations.** In the following days, increase to 200 repetitions.

FREQUENTLY ASKED QUESTIONS
(PELVIC FLOOR TRAINING)

Q: **What can I do if the juggling ball hurts?**

A: Start off without the juggling ball. Sit on a chair as described above. Place your middle and index fingers under your sitting bones. Push together your sitting bones with your fingers and repeat this exercise a few times. Then gently contract your sitting bones towards the perineum. Do you feel the tension around and between your sitting bones?

Q: **How often should I practise?**

A: Practise 10-15 minutes a day, 3-5 times a week.

Q: **What should I do if I get a burning sensation?**

The magic word is softer, softer, softer! Get lazy. The more relaxed you are when training your pelvic floor, the better. Tense your muscles so gently that you can only just sense that you are doing anything at all. Should the burning persist, take a day's break. Begin again right from the start until you can do it without the burning sensation.

Q: **I feel nauseous, why?**

A: The pelvic floor is a real powerhouse. It interacts with your stomach, legs, back and your internal and external genitalia. When rousing and actively treating dormant body areas, this activation can cause new and sometimes unpleasant body sensations. Probably, you are tensing your pelvic floor too much and are holding your breath. To start off, I recommend you practise without the juggling ball and only for 2 to 3 minutes. Let your breath flow gently and take care to keep a relaxed posture. Only increase your exercise time after a few days. When you are ready, practise with the juggling ball. Be good to yourself and your body and take your sensations seriously.

MAKE FRIENDS WITH YOUR PELVIC FLOOR

The following exercises have been chosen carefully. Take lots of time to do the exercises and give them your full attention. You will be more successful if you only do one exercise and do it very accurately, gently and carefully than if you do all the exercises, but with too much tension.

With all the exercises, you need to take care that you remain totally relaxed in your entire body. So, also relax your jaw, forehead, stomach, bottom, back, shoulders, hands, legs, feet and toes. When you feel you are tensing up, stop the exercise and start again from the beginning. Even if you find one or another exercise exhausting, always look for a feeling of lightness within your whole body. Then you can be sure: you are doing it properly!

What you need for the exercises

- Train in comfortable clothes, ideally barefoot or in socks.

- Use a yoga mat or a soft carpet as a base. Blankets are usually too slippery and make a relaxed training session difficult.

- A juggling ball, bean bag or stress-ball, (vinyl covered, bean filled) with a diameter of 4 to 6 cm (1.6 to 2.4 in).

IMPORTANT TERMS

Perineum: it is located exactly between the entrance to the vagina and the anus. If you place your fingers against your perineum, you will feel that the area is made up of relatively firm but still soft tissue. When pulsating, you can sense a slight movement within the perineum.

Sitting bones (ischial tuberosity): you can easily feel these bones, when you sit on a chair with a hard seat. Commonly, they are known as sitting bones or as pair of sit bones.

Activate the pelvic floor: very gently contract the sitting bones towards the perineum. Carefully extend the gentle tension in all directions.

See also "The pelvic floor basket: this is how it works" page #43.

Crown: the highest point on the head, also called skullcap or roof of the head.

FOR YOUR NOTES

LONG BACK

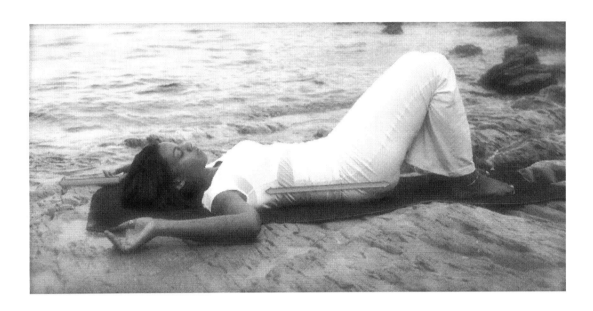

1 **Lie down comfortably.** Knees and feet are hip-width apart. Bend your knees so that your feet stand vertically under your knees.

2 **Imagine** you are breathing in through your right sitting bone. At the same time, move your right sitting bone towards the perineum. Let your breath flow towards the left iliac crest. In your mind, breathe out through the left iliac crest and relax, release your pelvic floor. Now breathe in through your left sitting bone. At the same time, move your left sitting bone towards the perineum. Imagine sending your breath towards your right iliac crest. Breathe out through your right iliac crest. Relax your lower back and pelvic floor. Do this exercise 10 times for each side.

This is what you should avoid:

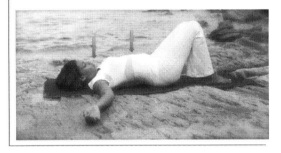

3 **Move your sitting bones** towards the floor. This will induce your pelvis to form a slight hollow back.

4 **Gently contract** the sitting bones towards the perineum. Immediately, but gently and with minimal strength, stretch the spine between perineum and crown (the highest point on your head).

This will pull your pelvis out of the hollow back position. You should neither be in the hollow back position, nor should you press your lower back into the floor. Link the tension from your perineum towards the front with the pubic bone, towards the back with the coccyx.

5 **Very gently, stretch your spine** a little more. Grow a tiny bit every time you breathe out. Your back feels very long and relaxed.

6 **Gently stretch your shoulders** to the sides and gently lower them backwards and downwards.

This is what you should avoid:

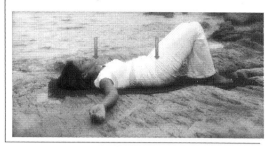

7 **Pulsate in your pelvic floor**, be really, really gentle. 100 pulsations.

GENTLE BACK ARCH

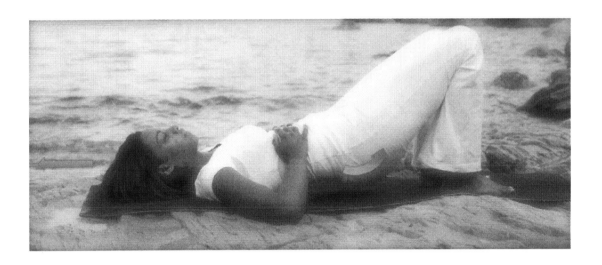

1 **Lie down comfortably.** Your feet should stand vertically under your knees. Knees and feet are hip-width apart.

2 **Activate your pelvic floor** by softly contracting the sitting bones towards the perineum. Relax your spine lengthwise, vertebra by vertebra. Gently stretch your shoulders to the sides and relax.

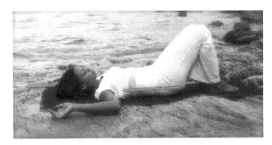

(Basic for this exercise is „long back")

3 **Curl your pelvis:** move your sitting bones towards the back of your knees; your bottom remains totally relaxed.

4 **Lift your pelvis** two centimetres (one inch) off the ground.

5 **Gently pulsate** in your pelvic floor. Every time you tense your pelvic floor, move your sitting bones a little more in the direction of the back of your knees. Curl your pelvis even more.

6 **While pulsating,** your bottom should remain as soft as custard and relaxed. Your stomach is relaxed, your shoulders are relaxed, your jaw and forehead are relaxed. Find the lightness in the exercise.

LOTUS FLOWER

1 **Lie on your back.** Place the soles of your feet against each other. The outer edge of your feet and your heels are touching. Stretch your back. Slightly curl your pelvis so that the length of your spine gently rests on the floor.

2 **Lift your heels** three centimetres (1.2 in) off the ground, the soles of your feet still remain together, your toes still touch the ground. Strongly press together your heels and the outer edges of your feet. This activates the inner layer of your pelvic floor. Your bottom, your lower back and your back remain relaxed and still. Release, press, release, press, release. 50 times.

3 **Press your heels together** again. Do you feel the slight tension at the back of your legs, the pull, the tension around your sitting bones? Take up the tension around the sitting bones: simultaneously press together your heels and pull your sitting bones towards the perineum. Release your heels, release your sitting bones. 50 times.

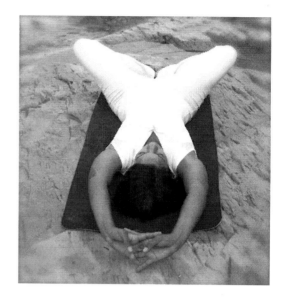

4 **Train with your breathing rhythm:** every time you breathe in, push your heels together. At the same time, gently pull the sitting bones towards the perineum. Every time you breathe out, release the pressure on your heels, relax your pelvic floor.

5 **Channel your breathing:** imagine breathing in through your perineum and let your breath flow up your spine towards your head. Breathe out through your crown, the highest point of the head.

PRONE POSITION

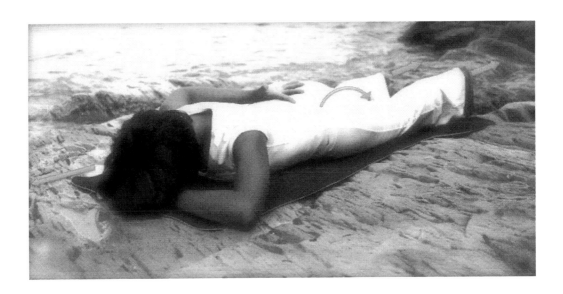

1 **Lie on your stomach,** legs hip-width apart, feet erect. Loosely place a hand on your bottom. Your forehead lies on your other hand. Relax your shoulders outwards and downwards.

2 **Activate your pelvic floor** by contracting the sitting bones towards the perineum. Your bottom remains soft and relaxed! If you tense your bottom, you will feel a slight movement under your hand. Take care that the hand on your bottom remains completely motionless.

3 **Move your sitting bones** towards the back of your knees – your lower back becomes long and relaxes. Your bottom remains relaxed.

4 **Stretch your spine:** in your mind, link your perineum with your crown (highest point on your head) and gently stretch.

5 **increase of difficulty** (optional): In turns, push your sitting bones towards your heels: pull your right sitting bone towards your perineum and push towards your heel, release. Pull your left sitting bone towards your perineum, push towards your heel, release. Right, left, right, left. Allow plenty of time for this exercise. You do not need to become a "pelvic floor expert" on the first day. This exercise will help you to relax your bottom while tensing your pelvic floor – something most women find very difficult.

Important: your bottom remains relaxed the entire time!

BREATHING PELVIC FLOOR

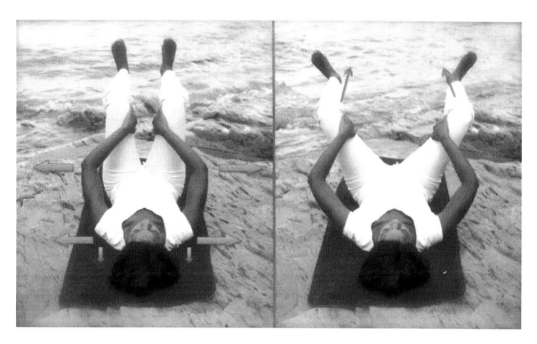

Take care to breathe in and out gently when doing this exercise. If you breathe in too deeply, you may take in too much oxygen and get slightly giddy. So, adapt the exercise to your breathing, not the other way round.

1 **Lie on your back.** Place your feet on the ground. Activate your pelvic floor by contracting the sitting bones towards the perineum. Link the tension with your stomach and back. Form the "pelvic floor basket". Carefully relax your back lengthwise, vertebra by vertebra. Gently stretch your shoulders sideways and downwards.

2 **Lift one leg after the other.** Bend your legs; right angle in your hips, right angle in your knees. Tighten your feet, energy in your heels: push away your heels without moving your legs.

3 **Loosely hold** the inside of your thighs with your hands.

4 **Every time you breathe in,** increase the tension in your pelvic floor.

5 **Every time you breathe** out, release the tension. Slightly spread your legs.

6 **Breathe in, activate the pelvic floor.** Breathe out, relax the pelvic floor. Spread your legs a little more.

7 **Spread your legs a bit more** with every breath. As far as your hip joints will allow.

8 **Stay in this position** for 2 to 3 breaths. Then close your legs, relax your pelvic floor.

9 **Relax for a moment** and repeat the exercise twice.

PELVIC EIGHT

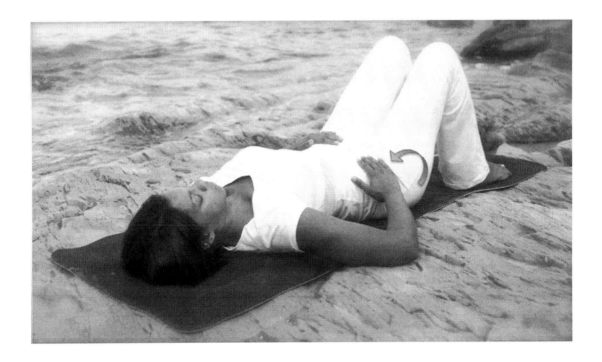

1 **Lie on your back.** Place your feet on the ground, knees and feet hip-width apart. Place your hands on your hip bones.

2 **Activate your pelvic floor:** move your sitting bones towards the floor to form a slight hollow back. Contract your sitting bones towards your perineum, then move out of the hollow back position immediately and stretch your back vertebra by vertebra. Link the tension in the perineum towards the front with the pubic bone, towards the back with the coccyx.

3 **Strongly pull your right sitting bone** towards your perineum, then push towards your heel.

4 **Pull your left sitting bone** towards your perineum and push towards your heel.

5 **In turns**, push your sitting bones towards your heels. Right, left, right, left.

6 **increase of difficulty** (optional): The movement is small and subtle. Move your sitting bones in little circles: towards your heels, towards your knees, towards your stomach. You can feel your pelvic bone under your hands. Move like a lying eight.

STEP 3
RELAX!

This is what you will learn in the third step:

❖ You will learn how to consciously relax.

❖ You will learn how to do gentle muscle relaxation (PMR).

❖ You will learn relaxing breathing exercises.

Contents

Today's performance-oriented way of life is highly stressful. We are constantly ready for action, we work, we study, our leisure time is full to bursting, and we hardly set aside a minute to relax. Many people find it difficult to "recycle" spent energy and to recharge their batteries.

This lack of balance in our energy store causes extreme wear and tear and weakens our potential. The consequences: tension, muscle pain, tiredness, exhaustion, headaches, indigestion, difficulty in concentration, mood swings etc. Extreme consequences of stress can even be depression, irritable bowel syndrome, panic attacks and burnout.

What happens when we are stressed?

A look into the ancient past: in primeval times, the human body was designed to release huge amounts of energy when stressed. Prehistoric man solved problems by fleeing, fighting or by playing dead. After a flight or a fight, he lay down and rested. Today, nobody can afford to have a nap after a tiresome meeting, and you simply cannot be seen getting out a pillow and putting up your feet after dealing with a difficult customer. But this way, these natural balance mechanisms are severely disrupted. We overexert ourselves more and more. Often, we also only sleep very little during the week. Thus our natural regeneration phases become too short to be able to stand our daily dose of positive stress.

Relaxation therapy is an effective method of regaining balance between stress and relaxation, for example with autogenic training, yoga, breathing exercises etc. Another method is progressive muscle relaxation (PMR), developed by the American physician Edmund Jacobsen. If practised regularly, it enables you to regenerate and unwind in a short space of time.

PROGRESSIVE MUSCLE RELAXATION

Progressive muscle relaxation (PMR) is very easy to do, and it is a method that you can learn and do by yourself. I will introduce you to a simplified version of PMR, which also incorporates the pelvic floor and which is consequently ideally suited to combat conditions such as vaginismus and vulvodynia. It will take full effect after approx. six to eight weeks. During this time, you should do one run-through every day – this will only take four to eight minutes.

Preparations:

1 Empty your bladder.

2 Sit or lie down comfortably. Make sure you will not be disturbed.

3 Preparatory exercise: make a loose fist. Pause (2 seconds). Build up a slight, pleasant tension. Hold this tension for two breaths. When you next breathe out, slowly and carefully release the tension, slowly open your hand again. Pause for one to two breaths. Repeat the whole exercise. Be sure to tense your hand so gently that you can only feel it in your forearm. If you can feel the tension in your upper arm or even in the back of your neck, you are doing the exercise with too much power.

Guidelines for practising PMR

- **Be as relaxed** as possible when doing PMR. Start off really softly, with minimal strength. Then, very carefully, build up a slight, pleasant tension. Hold this tension for two to three breaths and release the tension again, ever so slowly and gently. Repeat this twice with every part of your body.

- **Every exercise** follows this pattern. Step by step.

- **Take care** that the whole relaxation does not take too long so that you can really exercise every day. Only then will you feel the full effect of PMR.

- **The ending is always the same:** make a short and powerful fist with both hands, open the fist again. Take a deep breath and continue breathing normally. Also finish the exercise in this way if you are interrupted unexpectedly.

- **It is important** that you always do the PMR exercises in the same way. Only then can a kind of reflex arc develop. Your body learns: this is how to relax. When you are well practised, the mere thought of the exercise will make you feel more relaxed

PRACTISING PMR

1 **Close your eyes**, calmly breathe in and out through your nose.

2 **Loosely make a fist** with both hands, without any effort at all. Pause. Build up a slight, pleasant tension. Hold it for two to three breaths. When you are breathing out, gently release the tension, open your hands again. Short pause. Repeat.

3 **Gently move the tips of your shoulders** towards the floor, push the back of your head into the floor, push away your crown (highest point on your head). Build up a slight tension. Hold it for three seconds. Release the tension when breathing out. Pause. Repeat.

4 **Slightly raise your eyebrows.** Build up a slight, pleasant tension. Hold it for two to three breaths. Gently release when you next breathe out. Pause for two seconds. Repeat.

5 **Gently press together your lips,** your teeth, press the tip of your tongue to the roof of your mouth. Build up a pleasant tension, hold it for three seconds. Release the tension when breathing out. Short pause and repeat.

6 **Move your chin** slightly towards your chest, move the tips of your shoulders upwards. Build up a slight tension, hold it for three seconds, gently release the tension when breathing out. Repeat after two seconds.

7 **Gently tense your stomach** (pull it in or stick it out, whichever works better for you). Build up a soft, pleasant tension. Hold it for two breaths, slowly release the tension when you next breathe out. Pause for two seconds and repeat.

8 **Gently move your lower back** towards the floor, contract your sitting bones, softly tense your bottom. Build up a pleasant tension and hold it for three seconds. Gently release when you next breathe out. Pause for one breath, then repeat.

9 **Tense your feet**, pull up your kneecaps/tense your thighs. Build up a slight tension, hold it for two breaths. Gently release when you next breathe out. Short pause and repeat.

10 **Make a quick fist**, take a deep breath and continue breathing normally, open your eyes, focus your attention back on the here and now.

Sarah, 42, Frankfurt on the Main

"When I started with the 14-day-programme, I was really impatient. I wanted to practise properly right away – for me that meant with the dilators. Admittedly, I learnt the pelvic floor exercises and PMR, like a good girl, but I thought we weren't progressing fast enough. When I was back at the hotel, I wanted to insert my finger, but it didn't work.

At the next session, Claudia asked me how I had practised. When I told her, I realised that I had left out the relaxation exercises. We then had a long chat about relaxation and stress. In the evening, I did the PMR exercises really slowly, and then I took lots of time to appreciate and consciously train my pelvic floor. Then I tried once more to insert my finger. I again took plenty of time. I had to relax repeatedly in between. Whenever I realised I was tensing up, I did another PMR exercise. My finger did not slip in easily, but bit by bit it went in further, until it was completely in.

This experience showed me how important relaxation is for me to exercise successfully. I never again skipped the PMR exercises at the start. And every day I panicked less and less about practising. Even now, after really having beaten vaginismus, I still do PMR from time to time. It helps me to relax and to be a bit more laid-back about stress."

VIBRATIONS

Another form of relaxation is the "Vibrations" exercise. This may sound paradoxical, but it will help you to relinquish control over your body.

- **Lie down** on your back comfortably. Place your feet on the floor, close to your bottom. The inside edges of your feet are touching.

- **Spread** your legs a little.

- **Find a position** in which your legs shake or vibrate slightly.

- **Breathe** gently and calmly.

- **When the vibrating stops**, spread or close your legs a little, until they start vibrating again.

- **Stay** in this position for approx. 10 minutes.

step 3:

PRACTISING PMR

FOR YOUR NOTES

STEP 4

DISCOVER YOURSELF

This is what you will learn in the fourth step:

❖ You will come to know the female anatomy better.

❖ You will look at your "intimate face".

❖ You will touch yourself and overcome negative feelings that certain touches may trigger.

Contents

MAKING CONTACT

Whether they suffer from vaginismus or not, most women do not know their private parts really well. This chapter is all about getting to know and love your genital area.

You can do this exercise in comfortable clothing. Lie down comfortably, place your feet on the floor. Take 5 to 10 connected breaths. Direct your attention to your pelvic floor.

1 **Imagine breathing in through** your right sitting bone. Simultaneously pull your right sitting bone towards the perineum. In your mind, let your breath flow towards the left iliac crest. Imagine breathing out through the left iliac crest. Relax your pelvis, lower back and pelvic floor. Change sides with every breath. 5 times per side.

2 **Breathe in** through your right sitting bone and towards the perineum. In your mind, send your breath towards your left costal arch. Breathe out through your costal arch, let your ribs sink really gently, relax your pelvic floor. Breathe in through your left sitting bone, breathe out through your right costal arch. 5 breaths.

3 **Imagine breathing in** through your right sitting bone. Simultaneously pull your right sitting bone towards the perineum. Send your breath to your left shoulder. In your mind, breathe out through your left shoulder, relax your shoulder and pelvic floor. Change sides with every breath.5 times per side.

4 **Slightly spread your legs**. Place a hand on your genital area. The ball of your hand lies on your pubic bone, the fingers at the entrance to your vagina, the middle finger touches your perineum. The other hand lies on your stomach.

5 **Breathe in softly** and silently though your nose, open your mouth a little, breathe out with a quiet "aaah". Imagine you are breathing in and out through your perineum. Let your breath come and go. Let yourself fall a little more every time you breathe out, until you feel as light as a feather and totally relaxed.

A LITTLE ANATOMY

The female genitalia look as varied as the women themselves. The colour and texture of clitoris, labia and the perineal area can be very different.

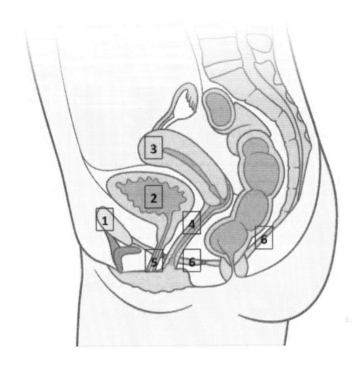

1 pubic bone
2 urinary bladder
3 womb/uterus

4 vagina
5 urethra
6 pelvic floor

➡ more details page #126

LABIA

The *outer labia* (labia majora) are located around the entrance to the vagina. Directly underneath runs the delicate muscle of the outer layer of the pelvic floor. Generally, the outer labia are hairy and slightly darker then the surrounding skin and less touch-sensitive than the inner labia.

The *inner labia* (labia minora) are hairless. They can be meaty and short or somewhat elongated so that they are

64

longer than the outer labia. The inner and outer labia are both very smooth, shiny and reddish or brown on the inside. The insides are full of sweat and oil glands as well as many nerve endings that make the labia very touch-sensitive.

Clitoris

Most people consider the outer, visible part – the clitoral glans – to be the clitoris. However, the clitoris is larger and connected to the pelvic floor muscles.

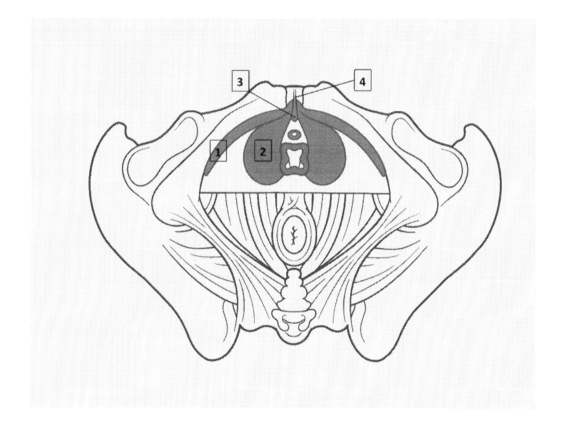

1 clitoral glans
2 clitoral body

3 clitoral crura
4 clitoral bulbs

➡ more details page #127

In all, the clitoris consists of four parts:

The clitoral glans (glans clitoridis), also called love button, can be very different in shape and size. It is highly touch-sensitive and therefore should only be touched or stimulated carefully.

The clitoral hood (praeputium clitoridis) covers the clitoral glans completely or partially and protects it from external irritation.

The clitoral body or shaft (corpus clitoridis) extends inwardly. It is palpable and between 0.5 and 4 centimetres (0.2 to 1.6 inches) long.

The two clitoral crura (crura clitoridis) make up the invisible part of the clitoris. They run deep within the clitoral body, along the pubic branch and to the sitting bones. Each crus is approx. 7 to 8 centimetres long. The outer layer of the pelvic floor muscles (musculus ischiocavernosus) runs directly above them. They are equally connected to the superficial transverse perineal muscle.

The clitoris serves no other purpose than to give pleasure and induce sexual arousal. Together with the urethral sponge, the anterior third of the frontal vaginal wall and the inner labia, it makes up a functional unit for sexual arousal.

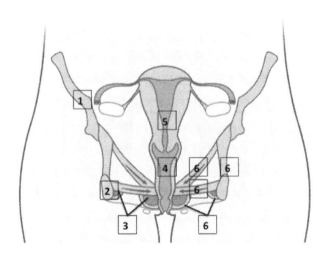

1 pelvic bone
2 sitting bone
3 erectile tissue of the clitoris

➡ more details page #128

66

4 vagina
5 womb/uterus

Vagina

The vagina is a highly elastic and muscular tube, which is lined with a mucous membrane. When not aroused, it is approx. 7 to 12 centimetres (2.7 to 4.7 inches) long. The anterior third of the vagina is surrounded by pelvic floor muscles, the inside is smooth, soft and warm. Usually, the vaginal walls lie close together. When aroused, the vagina widens. It becomes softer, wider and deeper so that it can easily accommodate a penis. The anterior (front) vaginal wall is more sensitive than the posterior (rear) vaginal wall. The anterior vaginal wall is connected with the urethral sponge – this area is also called G-spot.

The *G-spot* lies in the anterior vaginal wall, near the entrance to the vagina, and is connected to the urethral sponge. The G-spot tissue is rough and features longitudinal grooves. There are a great number of nerve endings on the G-spot area, which make it very touch-sensitive. The G-spot tissue holds numerous blood vessels, glands and channels as well as an enzyme that can also be found in similar form in the male prostate. That is why it is often referred to as the female prostate. When aroused, the G-spot swells. An orgasm in this condition is a much more intense experience and is often called "vaginal orgasm". Many women excrete a fluid when climaxing

6 pelvic floor

– so-called female ejaculate. As this secretion is expelled via the urethra, many women feel as if they were urinating when reaching their orgasm; however, this is not the case. The G-spot should be touched gently, especially if the woman is not aroused. This area is often pressure-sensitive and painful – especially in women who suffer from vaginismus and vulvodynia. If a woman is aroused, touching the G-spot will intensify her feeling of pleasure, and it becomes less pressure-sensitive.

By the way: the G-spot is named after the man who "discovered" and first reported about this highly erogenous zone, Dr. Gräfenberg.

The *A-spot* is also located in the anterior vaginal wall, between the G-spot and the mouth of the uterus. Its tissue is smooth and does not differ in texture from the rest of the vaginal wall. Stimulating the A-spot helps lubricate the vagina and intensifies the orgasm "deep within". This is also sometimes referred to as "uterine orgasm".

Uterus

The uterus or womb is a pear-shaped hollow organ consisting of muscles. It lies directly above the urinary bladder in the centre of the pelvis. The mouth of the uterus protrudes slightly into the vagina and is palpable through the vagina. When a woman is strongly aroused, the uterus retracts into the abdominal cavity, while the vagina becomes deeper/longer (12 to 20 centimetres / 4.7 to 7.9 in). When the mouth of the uterus is touched during sexual arousal, the uterus contracts. In case of a "uterine orgasm", it pulsates rhythmically.

THE MIRROR EXERCISE – LOOKING AT YOUR PRIVATE PARTS

You look at your face in the mirror every day. When you brush your teeth, when you put on your makeup, every time you are in the bathroom. You surely like your face. Perhaps there are also areas you do not like quite as much. Either way, you are well acquainted with your cheeks, your nose, your forehead, your mouth your chin.

And what about your genital area? Do you know this part of your body just well? Most women answer "no" to this. Many neither know the colour nor the size of their labia, their clitoris or their clitoral hood. Get to know one another. You private parts will become more familiar, and you will also find it easier to like your genital area. This mirror exercise will make it easier for you to perform the subsequent steps. But it will also simplify the vaginal training, the training exercises involving the dilators. Repeat the mirror exercise every so often, even when you have already started with the vaginal training. You will notice that any sense of shame will gradually subside, the more you become friends with your genital area.

- Do the mirror exercise when you have plenty of time to yourself. Switch off your telephone and mobile and make sure you will remain undisturbed for the next hour.

- Use a hand mirror for this exercise. Sit down comfortably so that you can see your genital area well with the help of the mirror. Support your back with a cushion.

- Spread your legs a little. Have a good, long, calm look at your genital area.

- What does your genital area look like? Which colour are your labia? What size is your clitoris, which shape is your clitoral hood? Do you like the look of your genital area, or are you disgusted? Look at yourself with loving affection! Smile. Smile your most beautiful smile. Your genital area is a part of you and incredibly beautiful. Learn to love it. And remember – your partner loves it, too.

- Gently pulsate with your pelvic floor muscles. What do you see? Do you see how your perineum and the area between your sitting bones slightly contract and curve inwards?

- Touch your labia. Gently pull your labia to the sides. Can you see the entrance to your vagina? Which colour is the entrance to your vagina? Pale pink or deep red? What do you feel? Curiosity? Fear? Nervousness? Calmly breathe in and out through

your nose and relax. Make friends with your genital area.

Repeat this exercise as often as you like, ideally daily. You will get to know one another quickly, and you are sure to get used to the sight of your genital area. Always look at your genital area with loving eyes. Learn to like it, or better still: love your genital area!

TOUCH WITH SENSITIVITY

Relax with a muscle relaxation or breathing exercise. When you are relaxed and calm, place your hand on your genital area, the ball of your hand on your pubic bone, your fingers pointing towards your perineum.

Do the exercise "Making Contact 62

1 **In your mind**, breathe in through your perineum. Simultaneously, gently contract your sitting bones. Breathe out through your perineum and relax your pelvic floor. Repeat this exercise a few times. Relax a little bit more every time you breathe out.

2 **When you are ready**, gently touch your right or left outer labium. Leave your finger to rest there for a moment.

3 **Massage** your entire outer labium in slow circles. Gently press point by point. Massage the whole entrance to your vagina like this. First the outer labia, then the inner labia, the

perineum and the entrance to your vagina. Let your breath flow, smile, remain completely soft and relaxed.

4 **If you like**, you can do this exercise with some lubricant. This will make every touch a little gentler and pleasanter. Take 10 to 15 minutes. Finish the exercise by pulsating a few times with your pelvic floor. What do you feel? Were you in pain? If yes, where? Repeat this exercise again and again, until you feel completely at ease and you no longer feel any pain.

Mélanie, 33, Zurich

"I was absolutely terrified of the mirror exercise. Looking at my face in a mirror was alright, but that stuff down there was not even part of me. Then I was to insert a finger. I tried again and again, but it was impossible. The entrance to my vagina felt just as sensitive as my eyeball. When I touched myself down

there, it was as if I was stabbing myself in the eye. The sensation was unbearable. I was devastated. Angry about myself and desperately sad. I wasn't even able to insert a finger. After a few attempts, I wanted to break off the whole treatment. Then Claudia told me, I should try the exercise 'Touch with sensitivity'. To begin with, I was to merely touch and let my finger rest there for a moment, then end the exercise. And every day, I was to leave my finger there a little longer. Then I was to massage the area in gentle circles. For me, this felt a lot better.

I did this exercise a whole three months before I could tolerate my fingers down there and even find the sensation pleasant. When I managed at last, I was extremely relieved. We were all really surprised how well I then coped with the dilators. Two months later, I had completed the entire programme."

FOR YOUR NOTES

STEP 5:

GET INTIMATE – VAGINAL TRAINING

This is what you will learn in the fifth step:

❖ How to insert your finger. Your finger will give you feedback on tension and relaxation in your pelvic floor.

❖ How to desensitise your vagina and re-gain control over tension and relaxation in your pelvic floor.

❖ How to practise with the vaginal trainers. You will start off with the smallest dilator and practise in various ways, until you are able to insert the largest dilator easily and without pain.

Contents

You have already learnt quite a lot: you have gleaned plenty of information on vaginismus, you have tracked back your own vaginismus history, and you have faced up to your fears and difficulties. You have got to know your pelvic floor and can now consciously tense and relax it.

You have already regained a lot of control over your pelvic floor, you have looked at your genital area and can comfortably accept contact there.

All this has prepared you to go the next step: the training sessions with the dilators. But first, you will learn how to insert your own finger.

ALL ABOUT VAGINAL TRAINING

The effect of vaginal training

The training with the dilators will desensitise your genital area and your vagina. You will get to know new body reactions, and you will learn how to control your pelvic floor in a more targeted and conscious way, until it does the right thing at the right moment again. Your current reaction "Something is approaching my vagina – the pelvic floor tenses up" will be retrained into "If I want to insert something, my pelvic floor relaxes and my muscles allow me, for example, to insert a dilator". The aim of the vaginal training is not to stretch your vagina! Your vagina is very elastic anyhow.

When you practise, it is advisable to always follow the same pattern. This will help you to persevere and to make a habit of practising. The more used you get to practising, the easier it will become for you to practise regularly and in a relaxed way. In "All about vaginal training" I have compiled experience-reports and tips from lots of women, which will make

the training exercises with the dilators a lot easier.

VAGINAL TRAINER, VIBRATOR OR YOUR OWN FINGER?

The success of the vaginal training does not depend on the type of implement you use. Crucial for success, however, is that you feel comfortable with and have a liking for your aid of choice. Every form, every material has its pros and cons. Preferably, start the vaginal training with your own finger and then choose the aid that most appeals to you. You can, of course, also use several different vaginal trainers during your self-treatment. This can make the battle against vaginismus a little more diverse and pleasant.

Vaginal trainers are usually made of silicone, plastic, wax or glass. To help you decide which one(s) to choose, here a short overview of the properties of the most commonly used dilators.

Amielle Comfort

The Amielle Comfort vaginal dilator is probably the most widely used. The set comprises five dilators as well as a tube of lubricant. It is the cheapest set available, and in most countries your health insurance will pay for the costs if you have a medical prescription. The dilators are made of medically tested plastic and are, of course, free from plasticisers and latex. They are a little harder than many other dilators – so be especially gentle when practising to avoid any discomfort. But the hard material also has an advantage: it makes the vaginal training more effective, as you will learn more quickly to sense the increased tension in your pelvic floor muscles. This way, the pelvic floor will learn very swiftly to relax at the right moment. Should the transition from the fourth to the fifth dilator be a little difficult – many women find the difference in size challenging here – you can also use an intermediate-sized dildo, vibrator or vaginal trainer from another manufacturer.

Note:

The dilators "Amielle Comfort" or "Amielle Care" we use at the P6 Beck-enbodenzentrum [pelvic floor centre] are available as a set of five. Their smooth surface enables you to insert them gently. They are made of clinically tested material and are therefore quite safe to use. The set includes a tube of water-based lubricant, a handle and a discreet and convenient bag to store the items in.

Silicone dilators

Silicone dilators are anti-allergenic, skin-friendly, medically safe to use, non-porous and easy to clean (generally dishwasher-safe). They are a little softer than plastic or glass dilators, which makes practicing somewhat more pleasant. But often the pelvic floor takes longer to learn to relax, because it encounters less counter-pressure. Silicone quickly adapts to your body temperature, something that women who are sensitive to cold greatly appreciate. Silicone dilators can be bought separately in six to eight sizes, hence moving on from one size to the next is a little easier, as the difference in size is smaller. However, they are more expensive than the Amielle set. If you prefer silicone dilators, take care to choose a lubricant that is compatible with silicone or simply use a water-based lubricant.

Glass dilators

Glass dilators are highly aesthetic, almost works of art. They are very skin-friendly and are therefore especially suited for sensitive women. Glass dilators are incredibly smooth and are easy to insert. As they do not become porous, lubricants stay on for a very long time, which makes the vaginal training easier. Glass dildos and dilators quickly adapt to your body temperature and can be used both warm and cold.

Dilators by "Passion Glass" are made of medical hard glass and are, if used appropriately, shatterproof. For safety reasons you should, nonetheless, store your glass dilators separately, as they can get damaged if they clash. All glass dilators are carefully tested before shipped. They are dishwasher-safe.

Vibrators and dildos

Vaginal trainers in the form of dildos or vibrators are available in various shapes and materials. They are especially suitable if you are already somewhat experienced and are ready to insert slightly bigger vaginal trainers, as the smallest vibrators/dildos on the market are usually a bit larger than the smallest dilators.

Some women like dildos that are reminiscent of an erect penis. This can be helpful in the transition period from vaginal training to the first time you take in your partner's penis. Vibrators can also make the exercises a lot easier, as the gentle vibrations relax the pelvic floor muscles. Practising with vibrators while you are aroused will lubricate your vagina and make the tissue of your vagina and your pelvic floor both softer and more elastic.

Preferably invest in vibrators made of skin-friendly and tested materials, especially if you buy a soft one. These products often contain "plasticisers" which may contain harmful substances. Therefore, always watch out for phthalate-free rubber when buying dildos/vibrators. Soft dildos made from silicone are quite safe.

Vibrators, thanks to their gentle vibrations, can help with relaxing your pelvic floor muscles. To begin with, you can also use vibrators externally, as a kind of massager, to stimulate yourself a little. Inserting a vibrator or a dilator can be easier and more pleasant if you are aroused during you vaginal training sessions. When aroused, your vagina becomes softer, moister and more flexible: three advantages for gentle vaginal training.

Wax dilators

Some manufacturers offer wax dilators. These are not quite as slippery as plastic, silicone or glass dilators, which slightly hampers vaginal training. In addition, wax frequently has an irritating effect on the vaginal mucous membrane. In this case, the use of condoms is advisable.

From nature

Many women may find the thought of inserting vegetables into their vagina repulsive. Nonetheless: natural vaginal trainers like, for example, carrots, courgettes or cucumbers are extremely cheap and can be cut into any shape you like. However, they do not slip in and out quite as easily as plastic, silicone or glass dilators. To improve slipperiness, you can use condoms, which will also make the "DIY" dilators feel smoother. If you want to use vegetables without a condom, please take care to only buy organic products that are free from pesticides or other harmful substances.

Like with all vaginal trainers, you should use a lubricant with your vegetable.

You can, of course, also use your fingers as vaginal trainers. This method is especially suitable for when you first start training. However, the more advanced you become, the more difficult it will become to practise with your fingers. Inserting two fingers at once is not a problem. But three fingers may already pose difficulties. Your fingers are shorter that the vaginal trainers, so you will begin to tense up. Consequently, your pelvic floor also tenses up, and you will feel a burning and stinging sensation while inserting your fingers, making the whole exercise unnecessarily tricky.

THE OPTIMAL LUBRICANT

A good lubricant is essential for pain-free vaginal training. It facilitates inserting a finger and vaginal trainers, it increases the slipperiness of the dilators and moistens the vaginal mucous membrane. All this reduces friction and irritation of the vaginal mucous membrane – you will be able to practise more easily and with fewer hitches. Do not save on lubricants under any circumstances. Neither when buying nor when using them. But which lubricant is the best? You can decide for yourself, which lubricant you prefer. But take care that your lubricant is skin-friendly, tested, and, if possible, perfume-free to reduce additional irritation of the

vaginal mucous membrane, especially at the beginning.

Lubricants are available from pharmacies, chemists, supermarkets, online shops or from (women's) sex shops. Sex shops aimed at women tend to be well-equipped with lubricants, dildos and vibrators that are especially geared towards women's needs. We offer a range of tested lubricants on our homepage that are particularly suitable for vaginal training. All of them are condom-friendly and suitable for all dilators – also for silicone ones.

Silicone-based lubricants

Most women favour this type of lubricant. It has the best lubricity properties and is slippery for a long time without getting sticky. Silicone-based lubricants instantly adapt to your body temperature and have a silky texture. The disadvantage: they often stain. However, the stains can be washed out easily.

Silicone-based lubricants are a little more expensive than other lubricants; but as they can be used sparingly, the cost is balanced out in the long run. Should you use silicone dilators for your vaginal training or condoms to prevent pregnancy or sexually transmitted diseases, bear in mind to only buy lubricants that agree with silicone products. Some silicone-based lubricants cannot be used with silicone dilators or condoms.

Water-based lubricants

Water-based lubricants are the most widely used. They are really skinfriendly and do not affect the delicate vaginal mucous membrane. I recommend you use liquid lubricants, as these stay slippery for longer than lubricating gels, which dry out more quickly and may become sticky during your training session. To prevent unwanted bacteria from thriving, water-based lubricants contain preservatives. For women, who are sensitive to preservatives, a silicone-based or mixed lubricant may be better. Advantages of water-based lubricants: they are condom-friendly, can be used in conjunction with all contraceptive methods, do not stain and can be easily washed off with water. Water-based lubricants are also available in various flavours.

Vaseline and oils

Products such as baby oil, olive oil, vaseline or milking grease tend to be insufficiently slippery, interfere with your vaginal flora and do not really belong in your vagina. Especially oils and fats containing essential oils often cause irritations and may trigger allergic reactions. If you nonetheless prefer cooking oil, take care to use organically farmed products to avoid pesticides and other harmful substances. Oils should not be used in conjunction with silicone dilators and condoms, as they will become brittle and stop being effective.

Oil-based lubricants tend to be a little more slippery and skin-friendlier than pure oils. However, if you are sensitive to irritations, are allergic or frequently suffer from infections of your vaginal mucous membrane, you should give preference to silicone- or water-based lubricants. Like all oils, oil-based lubricants will stain your clothes, towels and bed linen and are difficult to wash out again.

Lubricants with effect

As varied as the base ingredients of lubricants are, as different are the effects you can achieve with certain additives:

- Warming lubricants that stimulate the blood flow
- Stimulating lubricants that support arousal
- Skin-regenerating lubricants
- Lubricants with various flavours

You should always test first, whether a lubricant with additives agrees with your skin or not. If you can detect irritations after application, stop using this product. Rebuild your vaginal mucous membrane with products containing lactic acid. These products are available from your pharmacy, or your gynaecologist can give you a prescription.

IDEAS AND SUGGESTIONS FOR VAGINAL TRAINING

Admittedly, vaginal training is no walk in the park and definitely not the most beautiful thing in the world. It is merely an effective steppingstone on the way to a broader sexuality. But you neither have to become a champion at vaginal training, nor does it have to become the centre of your life. Make it as easy and simple for yourself as you can. Create a pleasant atmosphere and conditions in which you know you can relax and practise in peace. Turn off anything that might interfere, such as your telephone, mobile or other means of communication. The more comfortable you are during training, the easier it will be for you to exercise with the dilators.

BE CREATIVE WITH SETTING UP YOUR PERSONAL COMFORT ZONE

How about taking a warm bath to relax? Or maybe you prefer soft lighting and candles? Or a fragrant oil burner with your favourite scent? Music can have a great effect on the mood and help with your well-being. Try different styles of music. Choose music that soothes you and puts you in a happy mood. This does not have to be ambient or New Age music. You can play soul, pop, classic, love songs or whatever you like. However, songs that put your in a melancholy or sad mood tend to be counterproductive. In short: just experiment and see what helps you best to remain calm and relaxed.

Take the practise sessions easy

It can, of course, be a great burden for you and your partner not to be able to have and enjoy a carefree sex life. The situation becomes nerve-wracking and can even lead you to raise doubts about your relationship or arouse fear that your relationship will go to pieces. However, your aim is not only to succeed in enduring a gynaecological examination or to insert a tampon. To go on a journey of discovery to explore your body and to reach a broader sexuality with your partner should also include sensuality and fun.

The training is hard enough. There are fears that need to be overcome. Be it fear of pain, fear of inserting something or fear of failure. Make your journey as pleasant and casual as possible. Inserting a tampon should neither cause distress nor a burning sensation nor pain. And it should definitely not be a big deal. If it were, where would be the advantage of the discreet, simple, odour-free, hygienic and safe way of handling your period? A gynaecological examination should be possible without fear and pain so that a regular check-up can become a matter of course. And last but not least: sex should be fun. Sex should be a sensuous delight. As a woman, you may and should crave sex and be free to feel attractive, feminine, delicate, sensual, erotic, luscious, happy or dominant. But, from time to time, you may also not feel like it or just yearn for cuddles or want to do nothing at all.

I do not want to be presumptuous here, but training with the dilators can be just as playful as eroticism, passion, a relationship, as being a woman, a lover, a friend. Perhaps you are keen to practise today, but not at all tomorrow – then take the day off and do something else that makes you feel good. See the training as a new aspect of your womanhood, your relationship. Approach it with curiosity and ease. Playful yet serious and with a generous helping of nonchalance.

Never hurt yourself!

The most important principle of vaginal training is: "Pain is a thing of the past, this is the start of a pain-free, easy-going life!" Vaginal training will be simpler and more successful of you can exercise when you are completely relaxed. Pain causes discomfort, fear and tension – your well-being and relaxation evaporate, your pelvic floor, stomach and legs tense up, the vaginal training hurts even more ...

A slight burning sensation or uncomfortable feelings towards the beginning of the training are normal. Most people are sensitive to new sensations, especially if painful experiences have been predominant in the past. This can quickly be perceived

as a burning feeling. The calmer, more relaxed and serener you approach the vaginal training, the less discomfort you will feel and the easier the training will be for you. That is why pain is a definite no-go!

How often?

The more often, the better. If you practise regularly, you will make a habit of training. Getting started will be a little easier every time. You no longer have to laboriously bring yourself to do a training session. The longer the gaps between the individual training sessions, the greater the chance that you are thrown back a step again and that it will cost you quite an effort to continue with the vaginal training.

Many women practise with dilators for months or even years – sadly often without making much progress. For these women, practising tends to become a huge emotional, mental and physical effort. Frustration and demotivation are the sorry result. The longer a woman practises in this way, the greater the "vaginismus" problem becomes, and the woman and/or the couple focus increasingly on the non-functioning part of their sex life. Passion withers. Anger, sadness and disappointment set in. Often, all sexuality, all erotic and tender (physical) feelings are blocked out. It becomes increasingly difficult to associate good feelings and experiences with sexuality. Do your training as swiftly as your personality and your lifestyle allow you to. It should really only be a stepping stone to your goals: to use tampons, to undergo a gynaecological examination without fear and pain, and to enjoy your sexuality in a new and care-free way.

The more frequently and regularly you train, the quicker you will progress and successfully beat vaginismus. You will be more and more successful with your training, and it will become increasingly easy to handle. Plan your training as carefully as a doctor's appointment or a meeting. Give yourself a timeframe in which you want to make tangible progress. If all the training becomes too much for you in day-to-day life, take one or two weeks off work and dedicate this time exclusively to your training.

For how long?

Take plenty of time for your vaginal training. Ideally, you should practise without time pressure and without important appointments at the back of your mind. You will be more relaxed and consequently more successful, when you have no appointments, even things like going to the cinema with a friend, after a training session. Take plenty of time for your vaginal training, especially towards the beginning.

How long an individual vaginal training session takes varies a lot from woman to woman. Some women merely take 10 minutes, others practise for 30 to 45 minutes. To begin with, you will take a little less time than

later, when you practise with larger dilators. Listen carefully to your body – then you will automatically practise "correctly".

Position

Choose the position you feel most comfortable in for the vaginal training. You do not have to lie in bed and on your back if this makes you feel uncomfortable. If you want to practise on the bed, you can also sit up a little and lean back, a supporting cushion in your back, bent knees and legs slightly apart. Or stretch out one leg, and spread the other one sideways. Perhaps you prefer to practise lying on your side, one leg slightly bent, the other bent and with the foot flat on the bed. Simply try what suits you best.

Or you make the bathroom your training ground. Here you can, for example, practise standing up, with one foot resting on the rim of the bath or the toilet lid. Or maybe you prefer practising in the shower or in the warm bath. This is also possible. If you choose to practise in water, be sure to use a silicone-based lubricant to make inserting the dilator as easy as possible. Water will dry out your vaginal mucous membrane, and with a water-based lubricant you will have difficulties inserting the dilator without problems.

No matter which position you choose for the vaginal training: spread one or both legs sideways a little. The pelvic floor is more relaxed that way, and inserting the dilator will be easier.

HOW TO STRUCTURE YOUR TRAINING

Ideally, you should practise four to five times a week. Set aside 60 to 90 minutes for each training session. Maybe your training will be much shorter or a little longer – you alone determine the duration of your training sessions. Set aside a generous amount of time so that you can practise calmly and without any stress.

Prepare

If you do not own a training box yet, now is the time to invest in one. Put everything you need for your training sessions into your *training box*:

- The Amielle Set with the dilators
- Lubricants
- Tissues
- A hand mirror
- Your notebook or your training diary
- Exercise instructions
- Juggling ball for pelvic floor training
- Possibly a towel

To ensure your pelvic floor can truly relax, go for a wee before starting your training session. If you have a full bladder, your pelvic floor is tensed, and inserting a finger or a dilator can be tricky. Give the exercise – for example "Inserting a finger" – another read trough. Perhaps you would also like to write down in your own words, what you will do in your practice session. Visualise what you can do if you run into difficulties or feel discomfort when inserting a finger or dilator. For example, when you tense up or get a burning sensation.

Your training sessions should always run according to the same pattern:

1 First, progressive muscle relaxation, approx. 7 to 10 minutes.

2 Then, pelvic floor exercises, approx. 10 to 15 minutes.

3 Possibly mental training, 5 minutes.

4 Only then start practising with your finger or dilator.

FOR YOUR NOTES

INSERTING A FINGER

When you practise with your own finger, this has a similar effect as biofeedback. You not only feel the "sphincter" itself, but you can also sense the pelvic floor all around your finger. This experience is a great help in learning to appreciate the pelvic floor even better. Your own finger will then, so to say, give you feedback on whether you are tensing or relaxing your muscles around your vagina.

Difficulties you may encounter when training with your own finger:

- A sense of shame. Your vagina belongs to you just as much as your finger does. Your finger is the best way to feel the angle, pressure and speed of insertion. In addition, you feel how soft your vagina is, how strongly you are tensing your pelvic floor muscles and what it feels like when you relax them.

- You are afraid to hurt yourself or to introduce germs into your vagina. Cut your fingernails short. If you like, use a condom. That way you can protect yourself from injuries, bacteria, viruses etc.

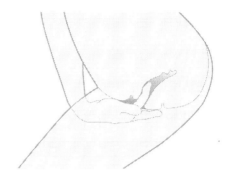

THIS IS HOW TO INSERT YOUR FINGER

1 **Lie down comfortably** and practise progressive muscle relaxation.

2 **Pulsate your pelvic floor muscles** approx. 200 - 300 times in total. If you are unsure, sit down on your juggling ball. If you are already well acquainted with the pelvic floor exercises, choose one or two of them. For example "Lotus flower" and "Gentle back arch". Always pulsate as softly as possible.

3 **Place your hand on your genital area**, the middle or index finger on your perineum, and breathe in and out through your pelvic floor 5 to 10 times.

4 **Massage your labia** and the entrance to your vagina with a lubricant. (See exercise "Touch with sensitivity", page #68.)

5 **When you feel the tension** around the entrance to your vagina

dissipating, you are ready to insert your finger. Apply plenty of lubricant around the entrance to your vagina and on your finger. Place your index finger on the entrance to your vagina.

6 **Gently pull apart your labia** with the index and middle finger of your other hand. The entrance to your vagina becomes palpable and visible.

7 **Breathe in and activate your pelvic floor**. Gently contract the sitting bones towards the perineum. Release the tension when breathing out. Breathe in, gently pull the sitting bones towards the perineum, breathe out, release. Upon releasing the third time round, you gently insert the tip of your finger.

8 **Stay in this rhythm**. Breathe in, activate the pelvic floor. Breathe out. Release the pelvic floor muscles. The third time round, push your finger in a little further. Continue in this way until you have inserted your whole finger.

9 **Leave your finger inserted** for 2 to 5 minutes. Pulsate in your pelvic floor.

10 **Consider the following**: how does this feel? Is your vagina warm, hot, moist? How do you feel? Are you okay? Do you feel queasy, sick? Are you breathing? Are you relaxed?

11 **After a comfortable time**, slowly remove your finger. Gently push along with your pelvic floor.

12 **Pulsate in your pelvic** floor again 3 to 5 times, finish the exercise.

WHAT SHOULD I DO IF I GET A BURNING SENSATION OR I FEEL PAIN?

- Gently pulsate with your pelvic floor muscles until the burning sensation subsides.

- Relax your bottom, stomach and legs.

- Open your mouth slightly and breathe out with a 'haaa'.

- Take your finger out and begin again right from the start.

- Insert your finger really slowly – millimetre by millimetre.

- Massage the painful area veeeery gently or softly press your finger on it.

Linda, 36, Oslo

"I was so afraid to insert something. I was regularly overcome by panic. When I did the mirror exercise, I was so tensed up that the entrance to my vagina wasn't even visible. I was convinced I would never be able to insert something as large as my finger. I set aside over an hour for this exercise. On the second attempt, it worked without a hitch. My finger quite literally 'slipped' in. It didn't even hurt. I had to take the hand mirror to make absolutely sure that my finger was really inside!"

MENTAL TRAINING

Do you have difficulties staying relaxed while you are inserting your finger? You can allay these fears with the help of mental training. Athletes frequently use mental training to improve and perfect certain movements to become better at their sport.

HOW MENTAL TRAINING WORKS

1 **Relax with PMR** or with a breathing exercise. Sit or lie down comfortably.

2 **Visualise** minutely how you insert your finger. Imagine precisely how you apply lubricant, how you pulsate in your pelvic floor, how you breathe.

3 **Picture yourself successfully** inserting your finger – with ease and pain-free.

Other effective techniques to deal with fear or unpleasant feelings that may crop up during practise are: erase visions of horror, deconstruct ideas that inhibit you and activate or "anchor" feelings of success. Try out what works best for you personally, what helps you to progress. You are your best expert and you alone can successfully beat vaginismus!

How to delete visions of horror

1 **Like watching a film**, visualise an unpleasant situation in your mind's eye.

2 **Freeze** an unpleasant scene into a still image.

3 **Imagine**, how this very same situation takes a pleasant turn and "ends well".

4 **Place** a tiny version of this ideal into a corner.

5 **In a flash**, shrink your problem image.

6 **Simultaneously**, the positive image suddenly becomes larger. Fill your entire mental image with this vision.

Practise until the exercise works well.

How to deconstruct ideas that inhibit you

If you have trouble inserting your finger or imagining ever inserting a dilator, deconstruct this process into single steps.

An example:

You would like to insert your finger. The idea of inserting your finger makes you queasy. Your stomach convulses. This is the first step.

You place your finger at the entrance to your vagina. Your body reacts even more strongly. Your hands become clammy, you feel nauseous. You are scared. This is the second step.

You try to insert your finger. Your pelvic floor tenses up, your vagina burns and aches. Your nausea intensifies, you break off the exercise.

How to proceed

1 **Break down the process** into its individual parts. If you are afraid to insert something, examine the individual steps. What happens exactly? Which steps take place?

2 **Relax.** Watch your breathing.

3 **Imagine** (still relaxed) the first step.

4 **Focus** your attention on your inner calm, on your breathing, on being relaxed. Finish the exercise.

When you feel comfortable with the exercise, extend it by one step. Finish the exercise once again with a relaxed attitude. Run through the entire process bit by bit.

How to activate or "anchor" feelings of success

Imagine the following: you hear "your" song on the radio and automatically think of a very specific situation. All at once you feel the feelings from back then, and you suddenly become really happy or sad, depending on what you are remembering.

This song, which always makes you happy when you hear it, is called an anchor. You know this "anchor princi-

ple" very well: it works in the same way with your name. Every time you hear your name, you react to it. The doorbell, the telephone, certain smells or scents, photos etc. work in the same way.

You can also place an anchor deliberately. For example, you can attach positive, important feelings and properties to a ring. Every time you touch the ring, these feelings and properties are roused in you. The more often you consciously make this connection, the quicker and more effective this anchor will work.

1 **Sit down and relax**. Watch your breathing. Give yourself a few minutes to calm down completely.

2 Think **of a situation** in which you were highly successful. For example, when you passed an exam.

3 **In your mind**, release all the positive emotions you connect with this situation. What did you feel? Which qualities helped you to succeed? For example courage, perseverance, curiosity, eagerness to experiment? You have all these characteristics!

4 **Connect a movement** (for example pressing together your thumb and index finger) or an object (for example a piece of jewellery you always wear)

to these characteristics. Visualise your success properties as vividly as possible.

5 **Breathe in deeply**, then continue breathing calmly. End the exercise with a positive thought.

In difficult or depressing situations, you can do this movement or touch your piece of jewellery. This will activate all these positive characteristics in you.

HOW TO INSERT THE SMALLEST DILATOR

You have already successfully inserted your own finger. Congratulations! Now you will go a step further and insert the smallest dilator. The procedure is the same as when you inserted your finger. However, it will feel different from your finger. You will see: it is easier than you think.

Prepare

1 **Relax** with the progressive muscle relaxation technique.

2 **Perform** one or two pelvic floor exercises or sit down on your juggling ball. Very gently and in slow-motion, pulsate 100 to 200 times in your pelvic floor. Then, quickly and lightly, pulsate approx. 200 times.

3 **Moisten** your finger and the entrance to your vagina with lubricant. Insert your finger first.

4 **Take the smallest dilator** and stroke it across your genital area.

Inserting the dilator

1 **Moisten the dilator** and the entrance to your vagina with plenty of lubricant.

2 **Place the tip of the dilator** at the entrance to your vagina.Gently pulsate 200 to 300 times in your pelvic floor. In your mind, breathe in through your perineum. At the same time, gently pull the sitting bones towards the perineum. In your mind, breathe out again through your perineum. Simultaneously release the tension.

3 **Pull apart your labia** a little with the fingers of your free hand so that the entrance to your vagina becomes palpable.

4 **Very gently, activate your pelvic floor** 3 times: contract your sitting bones when breathing in, release the tension when breathing out. Breathe in, activate the pelvic floor. Breathe out, relax the pelvic floor. When you relax your pelvic floor for the third time, simultaneously insert the tip of the dilator. Remember: breathe out while you insert the dilator. Because, if you breathe in while inserting the dilator, the body tends to tense, which of course also affects the pelvic floor, which in turn tightens the vagina and makes inserting the dilator difficult or even painful.

5 **Stay in the breathing rhythm you chose.** Breathe in and activate – breathe out and release. The third time round, push the dilator in a little further. Continue in this way until you have inserted the whole dilator.

6 **Should you feel a burning sensation**, your sphincter (a part of the pelvic floor) is tensing up. Stay with the vaginal trainer exactly where you are. Gently pulsate with your pelvic floor. Breathe in and softly contract your sitting bones; breathe out and simultaneously release your sitting bones. Pulsate until the burning sensation stops; then continue in the same rhythm as before.

7 **Should you become scared**, concentrate on your breathing. Observe how the air flows in and out of your nose; do not change your breathing pattern. Concentrating on your breathing will take you to the moment. To the here and now. This will leave no room for your fear.

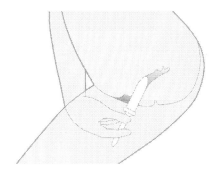

8 **Leave the dilator in your vagina** for a few minutes. Consider the following: how does it feel? Are you relaxed? How do you feel? Slowly pull the dilator out again.

9 **Gently pulsate** with your pelvic floor muscles two or three times. Finish the exercise.

10 **Before you start**, carefully read the above instructions several times. Possibly write down the individual steps again for yourself. Go through every step in your mind. Precisely visualise every teensy-weensy movement. How does it feel? How do you feel? What do you do if you get a burning sensation? What do you do if you suddenly get scared? And so on.

11 **Visualise yourself training successfully.** Mental training plus real training is the most effective strategy you can pursue. Imagine yourself practising with ease and that you succeed at everything without pain.

12 **Avoid negative phrases** with words such as "not", "no" etc. Form positive sentences. For example, change sentences such as "The training is not difficult, I feel no pain!

To "The vaginal training is easy and absolutely pain-free".

What should I do if I get a burning sensation?

- Gently pulsate in your pelvic floor until the burning sensation subsides.

- Relax your stomach, bottom, legs and pelvic floor.

- Relax your face. Slightly open your mouth, relax your jaw. Relax your forehead – smile!

- In your mind, breathe in and out through your pelvic floor. Relax when breathing out.

- Gently move the dilator back and forth, twist it or make circling movements with it.

- When nothing helps: remove the dilator, relax and start all over again.

This will help, when it gets difficult

- You feel a burning sensation or a slight pain when inserting the vaginal trainer. The burning sensation can occur when the pelvic floor tenses up. Hold the vaginal trainer calmly, yet with a little pressure. Gently contract your sitting bones and release them again when you breathe out. Gently pulsate in this way several times, until the burning sensation subsides.

- Change your position. If you are lying, stand up; if you are standing, lie down.

- Relax. Are your legs, bottom, stomach and face relaxed?

- Use more lubricant or use a silicone-based lubricant.

- Gently twist or rotate the vaginal trainer until the pain subsides.

- Concentrate on your breathing. Observe the way you breathe in and breathe out.

- Breathe out with an "aaah" or sigh when you breathe out. This releases tensions in your face, stomach, pelvis and pelvic floor.

- Visualise your pelvic floor. Picture how it relaxes. Use your imagination to conjure up an image that helps you. This could be, for example, an opening flower or melting chocolate.

- Breathe deeply in and out. Concentrate on relaxing your pelvic floor every time you breathe out.

- Many women find the vaginal training easier when they are aroused or after they have had an orgasm. When aroused, the vagina is softer, moister and more relaxed than usual.

- Look at the dilators every day. Pick them up. Stroke your genital area, the inside of your thighs, your pelvic area with them. This exercise reduces anxieties, lets the dilators seem smaller and desensitises your genital area. You are making friends with the dilators and are consequently less fearful of them. You will also find it easier to insert the larger vaginal trainers.

FREQUENTLY ASKED QUESTIONS (VAGINAL TRAINING)

Q: Do I have to insert the whole dilator on my first attempt?

A: No. It is sufficient to just insert the tip of the vaginal trainer when you first give it a go. You determine your own speed. You decide for how long, how quickly and how often you practice. I merely offer you points of reference, a guideline. But you are your own expert and know best what works for you.

Q: For how long should I practise?

A: Take plenty of time. You need approx. 30 minutes to prepare (relaxation, pelvic floor exercises, reading through the exercise). To begin with, practise 15 to 20 minutes with the dilator.

Q: How often should I practise?

A: Ideally, 5 times a week. But take good care not to go beyond your emotional limits and the time you can set aside for the training. Your training programme should fit into your day-to-day life. It should suit you – not the other way round.

Q: I want to finally insert the whole dilator, but I can only manage the tip. I'm always really disappointed then and close to breaking off the whole training.

A: Set yourself realistic goals. Break the step "insert the dilator" down into sub-steps such as "insert the tip of the dilator", "insert two centimetres (0.8 in) of the dilator", "insert three centimetres (1.2 in)" etc. Always only progress to the next step once you have successfully mastered the previous one. Also give your emotions time to keep up with the practise sessions.

Q: I cannot insert the dilator, although I desperately want to and am trying really hard.

A: Many women have to put a lot of effort into inserting the dilator for the first time. Some women are afraid to push or scared of injuring themselves when inserting the dilator. And sometimes the angle at which they are trying to insert the dilator is not quite right. Put the dilator aside for a moment.

Insert your finger once more. Make a note of the pressure and the angle at which you insert your finger. How do you insert your finger? Very gently, try inserting the dilator again. Practise with the mirror so that you can see what you are doing.

Q: I can insert the vaginal trainer, but taking it out again is painful.

This is very common.

"Inserting the dilator is very easy. But I get this really bad burning sensation when taking it out again. It's as if there is a vacuum and the pelvic floor muscles cling on to the dilator."

A: If you have difficulties removing the dilator, pull it out very slowly and push along a little with your pelvic floor muscles. Push very gently every time you breathe out – a little as if you were having a bowel movement. Sometimes it can also help to move the vaginal trainer back and forth or to rotate it slightly.

Q: I am on my period. Can I practise all the same?

A: Yes. Many women perceive their pelvic floor as softer during menstruation. Inserting the dilators is easier, because the pelvic floor is relaxed. If you suffer from pelvic pains or stomach cramps, skip the practise session. Remember: be good to yourself and to your body, and respect your personal limits and emotions.

YOUR TRAINING PROGRAMME

Proceed step by step as described above with every training session:

1 **Do the muscle relaxation** exercise according to Jacobsen, approx. 7 to 10 minutes. See PMR page #58.

2 **Choose two pelvic floor exercises.** In all, pulsate approx. 200 times during the exercises.

3 **Insert the dilator**; should you encounter difficulties, carefully reread the relevant passage in this book.

4 **Leave the dilator in** for a few minutes and pull it out again slowly.

ONCE YOU CAN INSERT THE DILATOR COMPLETELY, VARY THE VAGINAL TRAINING:

Leave the dilator inserted for a long time

Insert the dilator and leave it in your vagina for a long time. You can leave the dilator in your vagina for an hour and longer. But only leave it in for as long as you feel comfortable with it.

Repeatedly insert the dilator

Slowly insert the dilator 25 to 30 times. Take it out completely every time and insert it afresh.

Insert the dilator repeatedly in quick succession

Swiftly insert the dilator 25 to 30 times. Inserting the dilator quickly and repeatedly very effectively lowers the tension in the pelvic floor. The muscles learn to relax instantanously and you regain control over your pelvic floor. This form of exercise is also suitable for women who tend to suffer from cramps during the vaginal training.

Moving the dilator

Move the dilator back and forth several times. Insert the dilator, almost pull it out, insert it again, almost pull it out and insert it again. This form of vaginal training is particularly suitable for when you practise with the larger dilators and/or shortly before you carefully complete the final exercises together with your partner.

Practise all the variants until you can insert the dilator easily and pain-free. The dilator should "disappear", i.e. be almost imperceptible, before you move on to the next size. Reaching this goal can take just a few days or several weeks. Give yourself all the time you need.

HOW TO INSERT A TAMPON

There are many different types of tampons. With or without applicator, with soft rayon so that it slides in better, or simply made of cotton wool. You can get various sizes for days with a lighter or heavier menstrual flow. Use a tampon with applicator for this exercise. Take the smallest size available to start with. Once you can manage with the smallest size, you can also try out larger tampons.

Insert the applicator in the same way as you would the dilator. Then pull the applicator tubes apart a little and remove the tampon.

1 **Place the applicator** at the entrance to your vagina. Pulsate 200 to 300 times in your pelvic floor.

2 **Breathe in**, activate the pelvic floor, breathe out and release the pelvic floor. The third time round, insert the applicator a little.

3 **Continue in this rhythm** until you have inserted the tampon completely. If you like, you can practise while sitting on the toilet or while standing up, with one foot on a chair or the toilet seat. If you practise standing up, make sure your legs are spread. This position relaxes your pelvic floor muscles and makes inserting the tampon easier.

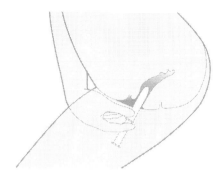

How to insert a tampon during your period

Pull the applicator apart. Insert the front end of the applicator completely, like you practised before. Push the back end of the applicator into the front end with your index finger. This will push the tampon into your vagina. Now slowly pull the applicator out again.

It is important that you insert the tampon quite deeply so that it comes to rest beyond your pelvic floor muscles. If the tampon is located in the outer third of the vagina, it will feel uncomfortable. It should feel as if the tampon had "disappeared"; then you have inserted it correctly. Pull the tampon out after approx. 2 to 4 hours or when it feels full. To remove it, pull the string and gently push along with your pelvic floor muscles. The time has come for removing the tampon if it slides out easily when you pull the string.

HOW TO CHANGE TO THE NEXT DILATOR SIZE

Stay with one size until you are able to insert the dilator quickly and easily on two different days.

Relax. Do your pelvic floor exercises as usual. Practise with your finger first. If this works well, insert the smallest dilator. If this also works without difficulties, take the second smallest dilator. Insert it in the same way you did the smallest dilator.

Like before, insert the second dilator step by step.

- Set yourself a realistic goal. It is sufficient to just insert the tip of the vaginal trainer, when you first give it a go.

- Increase the depth little by little, until you can insert the whole dilator – this can take several days or weeks.

- Try out the different variants of vaginal training: leave the dilator in for a longer period of time, insert it several times in a row or insert it gently and (almost) remove it again.

When you practise with the second, third, fourth or fifth dilator: always start off your training session with your finger, then with the first, the second, the third, the fourth, the fifth dilator. This acts as a kind of "warm-up" and will put you in the right mood for the vaginal training with the bigger dilators. If you feel confident

step 5:

and are sure you no longer need the smallest dilator, leave it out and start directly with the second dilator. It is, however, advisable to always begin with your finger. This way you can feel how your pelvic floor muscles are doing.Is your pelvic floor ready? Is it relaxed or a little tensed up? The step from the fourth to the fifth dilator ("Amielle Comfort") is often perceived as very large. To make this transition easier, you can purchase a silicone dilator, a dildo or a vibrator in an intermediate size. Especially in this phase, when you are already very confident in using the dilators, it is helpful to structure the training a little differently from time to time. Try inserting the dilators when you are aroused. Or practise with a vibrator, which will stimulate you with its gentle vibrations. Perhaps you would also like to practise with a soft penis-like (silicone) dildo to prepare for the partner exercises.

FOR YOUR NOTES

STEP 6:
PARTNER EXERCISES

This is what you will learn in the sixth step:

❖ How to, step by step, relinquish control to your partner.

❖ How to master the last steps together.

❖ How to insert your partner's penis into your vagina without pain.

Contents

You have completed all the previous exercises by yourself. Maybe your partner has supported you, celebrated successes with you. But what you have achieved so far has all been exclusively your doing. This will change with the partner exercises. You will need your partner. And your partner will need you. The success of the following exercises depends on your mutual willingness to communicate openly, to phrase needs sensitively and to respond to the other's needs. You now have to rely on your interaction as a couple.

The following exercises build trust. In your own pace, you will learn to slowly open up to your partner. You will relinquish more and more control to your partner.

Note: choose a contraceptive method you like before you start with the partner exercises.

SENSATE FOCUS – OPEN UP TO SENSUALITY

Over the last few weeks, you have concentrated a lot on your genital area and on successfully inserting your finger, tampons and the vaginal trainers. Sensate focus leads you away from your genital area and opens your whole body up to sensual experiences and "body communication" with your partner. Many couples enjoy being affectionate with one another without having to think about the dilators or about inserting something.

Guidelines for the exercises

The guidelines are not essential. They are simply there to give you an idea about how you can deal with the contact exercises. You can also agree on your own rules. But keep to what you have both agreed upon; this way you will create security and trust.

- Create a comfortable atmosphere.

- Take care you have warm, clean hands.

- In every exercise, each partner is once the giving, once the receiving person. If you like, you can both close your eyes.

- Talk as little as possible. Instead, talk about your feelings once you have completed the exercise. If a certain touch is unpleasant, do not put up with it, but address this immediately.

- Set aside at least 15 minutes for each exercise.

- Start off with "harmless" body parts, i.e. hands, head, shoulders, arms. Then proceed to the whole body. Your genital area comes last.

- This is not about sexual arousal, but about pleasant, sensuous touches. It is of course nice if you get aroused, but this is not the aim.

- Agree that neither fingers, nor the dilators nor the penis are to be inserted.

- Stay mindful and in the moment.

- Experiment with various types of touches. Slow and firm, gentle pats with your fingers, back of your hands, your hair ...

- If you like, experiment with different materials such as massage oil, body powder, feathers ...

Sensate focus: the hands

The giving person strokes the receiving person's hand. Take plenty of time. Stroke the palm, the back of the hand, every finger individually. Appreciate the different structures.

Sensate focus: the face

Gently feel the entire face and head of the receiving person: eyes, lips, nose, cheeks, ears, nape and so on.

Sensate focus: the rear of the body

The receiving person lies comfortably on his/her stomach. First, the giving person caresses the head, the nape, the shoulders, arms, hands. Continue down the back, to the bottom, to the back of the legs, to the feet. Leave out the inside of the thighs and the genital area.

Sensate focus: the front of the body

The receiving person lies comfortably on his/her back. First, the giving person touches the face, shoulders, arms and hands. Then the chest, the stomach, the front of the legs and the feet. For now, leave out the breasts, the genital area and the inside of the thighs.

Sensate focus: give the whole body a treat

First, the receiving person lies on his/her stomach. Caress the entire rear of the body (see above). This time, also include the insides of the thighs. The receiving person turns on his/her back. Caress the entire front of the body, including the breasts, the genital area and the inside of the thighs. However: for now, caress only and do not insert anything.

Sensate focus with dilators

Insert a vaginal trainer. You can use the smallest one to begin with. Repeat the sensate focus exercises. Observe: how do you feel when you are caressed or when you caress your partner and have something inserted in your vagina? Does your pelvic floor tense up again or can you relax and enjoy?

Should you have difficulties, practise again and again in different ways until you feel comfortable.

NATURAL BIOFEEDBACK

Insert your partner's finger

Prepare as usual:

* Relaxation.

* Pelvic floor exercises.

* Insert your own finger and the smallest dilator.

When you are ready, fetch your partner. If you like, he can already be with you while you practise. Show your partner how you practise. Explain to him how you breathe, how you actively use your pelvic floor and how you gradually insert your finger. Insert your own finger once again. Your partner places his hand on your hand and lets you guide his hand. He is to appreciate what kind of pressure you use to insert your finger. Also at which angle and how quickly you insert you finger. At no time does your partner push along; he only observes.

Swap over: now hold your partner's hand. Your partner allows you to guide him again. Your partner keeps the finger you want to insert rigid, immobile. Moisten your partner's finger with lubricant. Hold your partner's hand and insert your partner's finger little by little. Proceed in the same way as if you were inserting your own finer. Breathe in and gently activate your pelvic floor. Breathe out, release your pelvic floor and relax. When you breathe out for the third time, insert the tip of the finger while you are releasing the pelvic floor. Gradually insert your partner's finger in this way. When your partner's finger is fully inserted, leave it in your vagina for a moment. Pulsate in your pelvic floor. Give yourself and your partner some time to appreciate how this feels.

What to do in case of a burning sensation or pain:

When you feel pain, your pelvic floor muscles will tense up. Proceed in the same way as you did when practising with the dilators:

* Gently pulsate until the burning sensation subsides.

* Breathe calmly and steadily.

* Relax your legs, bottom, stomach, jaw and face.

For your partner

* Your partner allows you to guide him. At no point in time does he press or push along.

- Your partner keeps his finger absolutely still and rigid.

- Your partner gives you feedback. Can he feel the ring-shaped, muscular nature of your pelvic floor? What is the tension like? How does it feel when you pulsate in your pelvic floor?

- If your partner gives you exact feedback, it can be classed as a form of biofeedback. You feel differently than your partner. Maybe he can perceive a tension in your pelvic floor before you can feel it yourself. Or you can already relax your pelvic floor muscles a lot better than you think. Although this exercise costs quite a lot of effort to begin with, give it a try. It will be really worthwhile for you both: your partner will at last be included in your training process, and he will gain the feeling that he is needed. He can actively support and help you.

Your partner inserts his finger – under your supervision

- Swap over: place your hand on your partner's hand.

- He inserts his finger, step by step. You support him.

- Pay attention to your breathing. Breathe in and out calmly.

- Relax.

- Breathe in, gently contract the sitting bones towards the perineum, breathe out and relax.

PRACTISE WITH THE DILATORS TOGETHER WITH YOUR PARTNER

- Prepare as usual for the vaginal training. Together, create a comfortable, familiar atmosphere. If you want, do one of the sensate focus exercises first.

- Show your partner how you practise with the dilators. Pick up the smallest dilator.

- Your partner places his hand on your hand. Insert the dilator as usual.

- Let your partner feel how you insert the dilator.

- Your partner pays close attention to the way you insert the dilator. How quickly, at which angle, with how much pressure.

- Your partner's hand remains absolutely relaxed. You are in control of inserting the dilator.

- Take plenty of time. If your pelvic floor tenses up, relax. Breathe in and out calmly. Gently pulsate a few times with your pelvic floor muscles until you are relaxed again. Then insert the dilator a little deeper.

Your partner inserts the dilator – under your supervision

- Your partner holds the smallest dilator. Place your hand on his hand.

- Your partner's hand is slack and relaxed.

- Now gradually insert the dilator as usual.

- Your partner does not rush you, does not push along and leaves you in control of inserting the dilator.

Insert the dilator this way several times in a row. Once this works well, also insert the other dilators together with your partner in this way – until you can easily insert the largest dilator. If you get a burning sensation or feel pain, proceed in the same way as you would if you were practising on your own. Pulsate, breathe calmly, relax. You are ready to move on to the next exercise once you can insert the largest dilator together with your

partner – without pain, without tensing up.

Your partner inserts the dilator

- Prepare for the training as usual.Let your partner insert the smallest dilator. Agree on a stop sign; this way you will feel more at ease. Proceed in the same way as with the previous exercises.

- Your partner holds the smallest dilator, you place your hand on his hand.

- Your partner inserts the dilator, little by little. As always, take three breaths: breathe in, activate your pelvic floor; breathe out, simultaneously relax your pelvic floor. When you breathe out for the third time, your partner inserts the vaginal trainer a little bit.

Continue in this way until your partner has inserted the whole dilator. How do you feel? Are you able to leave your partner in charge? Are you relaxed? Is your pelvic floor relaxed? Repeat this exercise until you can, together as a couple, insert all dilators without difficulty.

FROM EXERCISING TO SEXUAL INTERCOURSE

Please remember: without some form of contraception, you may get pregnant when performing the following exercises. Please ask your

doctor for information on sensible contraceptive methods.

You have made it. You have reached an eagerly awaited step: you are saying good-bye to practising and hello to sex. It is an overwhelming step for you and your relationship, both emotionally and physically. You have learnt everything you need for this step: you have made peace with your genital area. You can insert your finger, a tampon and a dilator the size of an erect penis, completely pain-free and relaxed. You are ready to leave behind the most difficult steps and to enter into a new era of sexuality and, consequently, of your partnership.

Many women feel that inserting the penis is more natural than practising with the vaginal trainers. This feeling greatly facilitates this step. You will see, it is easier than you think: a penis is soft, warm, yielding and adapts to your vagina. Quite different from the cool, smooth and hard dilators.

Welcome the penis

First of all, your vagina will have to get accustomed to the penis. This approach will help you to remain relaxed, when you insert your partner's penis. Inserting the penis is neither the intention nor the aim of these exercises. These exercises are there to build trust, and your vagina will become acquainted with the penis. You will appreciate what a penis feels like.

- Together, find a position in which your genital areas touch.

- Gently take your partner's penis into your hand and guide it

towards the entrance of your vagina.

- Carefully caress your labia, clitoris, perineum and the entrance to your vagina with the penis.

Take plenty of time to appreciate the softness, the warmth of the penis. What do you feel? Are you relaxed? Are you breathing calmly? Experiment together. What does it feel like when your partner has an erection or when his penis is relaxed?

Expand the exercise:

Lie down comfortably.

Have your partner stroke his penis across your vulva through his movement. Again, penetration is not the aim of the exercise. You should merely make contact with the penis and get used to the emotions and feelings involved.

Position: Woman on top

- You have the absolute control over thrust, depth, angle etc. of penetration.

- You have eye-contact with your partner.

- This is an ideal position for the 'first time'.

- Disadvantage: your legs will tire quickly.

- Some women feel shame in this position

INSERTING THE TIP OF THE PENIS

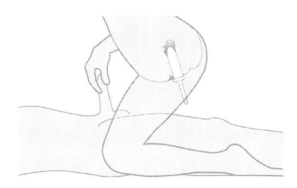

1 **Prepare as you would for the vaginal training**. Then insert the largest dilator. Change to the "woman-on-top" position. Your partner lies on his back, you kneel over him. His penis is in front of you.

2 **Moisten** his penis with lubricant.

3 **Stimulate** it, arouse it. Ask your partner what he likes. Your partner should now be able to hold his erection over a longer period of time without moving. For many men this demand is a real challenge. Support him with this task. Ask your partner what he needs to maintain his erection.

4 **Remove the dilator**. Now align your pelvis, the entrance to your vagina, with your partner's penis. Your partner can hold you around your waist to support you.

Slowly lower your pelvis until you can feel the tip of the penis at the entrance to your vagina.

5 **Gently pull apart your labia** with the fingers of your one hand. With the other hand, hold the penis.

6 **Pulsate in your pelvic floor:** breathe in, at the same time lightly pull your sitting bones towards your perineum; breathe out and simultaneously relax your love muscles. When you release your muscles for the third time, slowly lower yourself onto the tip of the penis. Gently insert one or two centimetres (0.5 to 1 inch) of the tip of the penis.

7 **Freeze in this position** for a moment. Calmly breathe in through your perineum, then breathe out again through your perineum. Pulsate in your pelvic floor. Appreciate what the tip of the penis feels like.

It may not feel all that great. It is a new sensation for you, a new experience. Give yourself time to get used to it.

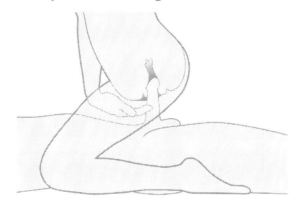

This may help:

- If you cannot insert the tip of the penis, insert the largest dilator once again. Leave it in your vagina for a few minutes. Veeery, veeery gently pulsate 100 to 200 times. Repeat the above steps again. And then insert the tip of the penis once more.

- In case of a burning sensation: you already know the tips from the vaginal training. Pulsate until the burning sensation subsides.

Massage tensed up areas with your finger. Breathe. Relax.

- You may need a few practise sessions before you can insert the tip of the penis. Do not lose heart. Persevere. Here, too, practise regularly and several times a week.

- How are you positioned? Often, the angle at which you are trying to insert the tip of the penis is not quite right. Adjust your position. To comfortably insert the tip of the penis, you may need to shift closer towards your partner's pelvis.

step 6:

INSERTING THE TIP OF THE PENIS

INSERTING THE WHOLE PENIS

Start in the same way as you did when you inserted the tip of the penis. First, insert the largest dilator. To begin with something you can already do with ease will build confidence in yourself and your body. You will once again realise that you are in control of your love muscles and that you can consciously tense and relax them.

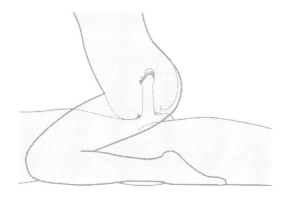

1 **Kneel** astride your partner again.

2 **Moisten** your partner's penis with lubricant when he is aroused.

3 **Pulsate** in your pelvic floor.

4 **Hold the penis** and insert the tip of the penis.

5 **Lower yourself down, step by step.** In the same way you inserted the dilators before. This step can take days or weeks.

6 **Give yourself** all the time you need.

7 **When you have inserted** the whole penis into your vagina, stay like this for a few minutes. Breathe calmly. Pulsate with your pelvic floor muscles. Allow your emotions. How does the penis feel? How does it feel when you pulsate? How do you feel?

8 **Finish** the exercise.

What do you need now? Listen to your inner voice and do what you need and what you would like best now. Talk to your partner. You are ready for the next step when you are able to insert the whole penis without pain or pelvic floor cramps on two separate days.

Move about

Congratulations! "Technically speaking" you have reached the end of the programme. In step 7 you will find tips on how to turn sexual intercourse from a technical procedure into a sensual, intimate encounter between two partners.

But first you will have to learn to allow movement.

Only you move

■ Prepare as usual.

■ Go into the "woman-on-top" position again. Completely insert your partner's erect and lubricated penis.

■ When you feel neither pain, a burning sensation nor cramps, start moving slowly. Should you get a cramp, stop moving. Pulsate until the cramp subsides. Only then start moving again.

You may find the movement unpleasant at first. Over time, when you have got used to these new feelings, it will become more pleasurable. Take all the time you need to arrange and integrate these new sensations into your life. Pulsate along with your pelvic floor: activate your pelvic floor when you move away from your partner. Relax when you completely lower yourself down onto him. This strategy will help you to manage any last cramps that may crop up. In addition, this will make you feel more comfortable and intensify your arousal.

Only your partner moves

■ Start in the same way as in the previous exercise.

■ When the penis is completely inserted, lift your pelvis slightly.

■ Now your partner moves his pelvis, pushing his penis deeper and pulling it back out again a bit.

■ Breathe calmly, flowingly.

■ Pulsate along in your pelvic floor.

Move together

Now it is time to start moving together: your pelvises both touch and move away from one another simultaneously; the penis remains in your vagina.

Pulsate in your pelvic floor again: activate when you move away from one another, relax when you come together again.

Find a common rhythm, adapt to one another.

These last steps can be emotionally overwhelming. Allow plenty of time for these steps. In the course of the following weeks, practise 3 to 4 times a week together with your partner so that you can get used to the new sensations.

FOR YOUR NOTES

STEP 7:
SEX AND MORE

This is what you will learn in the first step:

❖ From the technical procedure to a sensual encounter.

❖ Get to know your needs.

❖ Sex talk: speak to one another.

FOR HOW LONG SHOULD I PRACTISE WITH THE DILATORS?

You would like to chuck the dilators into a corner now and never use them again? Don't do it yet; cement your success first! Continue to exercise regularly with the dilators or with a vibrator/dildo in the course of the next two to three months. This way you will successfully beat vaginismus in the long run. Experience has shown that it may still be necessary to practise three to four times a week during the first month. After that, you can leave out one more practise session every week. Then continue to practise with the dilators once a week until you feel assured enough to completely drop the training sessions with the dilators.

The partner exercises are also very important. Do not overwhelm yourself with the thought: "We've made it. The rest will follow of its own accord." Give yourself time to develop a beautiful, pleasurable sex life. Continue to "practise" with your partner over the next two to three months. Continuing to describe any intimate encounters with your partner as "practise" will give you a few advantages:

* It is no big deal if it does not "work out" every once in a while.

* There is no need to pressurise yourself, and you are free from any sort of obligation to succeed.

* You may continue to practise gradually and with a clear conscience:first with the dilators, then slowly insert the penis and then move. Practise until you feel confident.

* Little by little you may and will be able to relinquish control and "let your guard down".

Over the next few weeks, set aside some time for the partner exercises three to four times a week. Go as far as you both feel comfortable with. You will be able to relax a little more every time. And the more relaxed you feel, the more open and susceptible you will be for sexual pleasure and arousal. You will encounter body sensations, but also emotions, that are new and unfamiliar for you. Roughly a third of all women initially find these new feelings unpleasant – but by degrees they perceive them as more and more exciting and fascinating. All these are important steps away from practising and towards sexual intercourse, which has not only become technically possible, but which you can now also consciously enjoy.

Congratulations – you have accomplished a brilliant emotional, physical and mental feat! Over the past weeks and months you have learnt a lot about yourself and your body. You may have been totally incapable of inserting anything into your vagina at the beginning of the programme. Now you can insert your fingers, tampons, dilators and your partner's penis. You can enjoy pain- and cramp-free sex.

However: some of you may ask yourselves: "Is that all?" Maybe you are technically able to have sex with your partner now, but you do not really feel any pleasure. The focus on "getting it in" may have let you forget the passionate side of sex. The moment has come to put the same intense effort you put into beating vaginismus into your relationship, into your sex life. Even today, many women (sub-consciously) think: "Once I've managed to get it in, everything will be okay."

Many women also say:

"I just want to get pregnant or at least be able to have sex so that I can feel like a woman.

I don't really care whether I have fun or not." I often get to hear statements such as these from women who have suffered from vaginismus for years. A pity. Sex and your sex life should be a fun and pleasurable experience. After all, it is the "most beautiful thing in the world".

Sex between two partners is the most intimate form of communication and sets a romantic relationship apart from deep friendship – we cannot be closer to a partner, both in the figurative and in the physical sense, than when we make love. Therefore, it is well worth to not only invest in your technique, but also in your passion.

ENJOYING SEX

Many women who have successfully completed the last step of my training programme "Vaginismus besiegen®" [beat vaginismus] ask themselves: "Is that all?" – "Is this really the most beautiful thing in the world?" Do not belittle your tremendous success with thoughts such as these! This would be counter-productive and could quash your motivation to continue on this newly discovered path of passion. It could dissuade you from exploring, playing with and enjoying your sexuality as well as your partner's.

It is a common misconception that the man merely needs to penetrate and everything is marvellous! Sexual intercourse stands for much more than a simple "in – out". Many couples are busy battling vaginismus for years and are so fixated on their problem of "it is impossible for us to have sex" that all intimacy and affection are lost. Because they are focussing so much on penetration, they forget that affection, spontaneity and fun are also part of the bigger picture.

When two people have just fallen in love, they want to get to know one another better. They spend lots of time together, they talk for hours on end, they discover what they both like and so on. But as soon as they are about to have sex, the getting-to-know-one-another phase is put on hold: it should and must work straight away.

Give yourself this period of getting to know one another, also and especially with regard to your sex life. Take time to explore your own and your partner's body and to appreciate one another in harmony. Find out what you like and talk about it with your partner. Create a sensual atmosphere in which you can both be intimate, tender, respectful and open to one another.

Fact: many women need a few weeks time before they feel that sex has turned from a mechanical act into a passionate and pain-free pleasure.

The following tips do not represent a comprehensive list! They are merely ideas and suggestions as to how to achieve a sensual, open sex life.

Have sex three to four times a week

Even if this may feel like a lot to begin with – consciously set aside this time for sexual intercourse with your partner. The more often you have sex, the more pleasant and more enjoyable it will become for you. Your body will get used to the new sensations. It will change, when you practise sex regularly. You will become wetter, penetration will become easier, you will become more relaxed and you will be able to relinquish more and more control and devote yourself to your partner.

Sexual arousal

Sensual sex is impossible without arousal. Your sex organs and your body need arousal. This is your body's way of preparing for sexual intercourse. When you are aroused, the colour of your sex organs changes, your vagina becomes wider, softer and moister. Your partner can penetrate more easily, you can both move more easily. Take plenty of time for a good long foreplay that arouses you both.

Tender gestures

Many couples lose interest when they have been battling vaginismus for years. Frustration sets in, and all feelings that are closely related to a sensual sex life are simply ignored. Often they are ignored so thoroughly that all affection dies. Consciously dedicate yourself to displaying affection again. Remember what you like about your partner. Rekindle a little romance. Take care to communicate lovingly. Build closeness and trust. Sex does not always have to entail sexual intercourse. There are many thousand other intimate, passionate, arousing little games you can play. You now have the freedom to decide.

Training the pelvic floor

You have got to know your pelvic floor quite well and learned how to train it. In one of the steps you have learned that the genitalia are closely linked with the pelvic floor. A well

and flexibly trained pelvic floor intensifies passion and orgasms. Therefore, continue training regularly or enrol in a professionally run class for pelvic floor exercise.

Masturbation

Discover your sexual preferences, wishes and needs. Masturbate every now and then. Only if you know your own body well, will you know what you like and what you don't like. The better you are at appreciating your erogenous zones, the easier it will become for you to feel passion together with your partner.

Sex talk: get talking

Couples who have beaten vaginismus together have another advantage: they can openly talk about things that other couples would blush to even think about. Please keep up this openness. Have the courage to openly talk to your partner about your preferences, fantasies and needs. Learn to tell one another openly what you would like to do. This may not be easy at first, but you will see that your partner will 'um' and 'ah' just as much as you. Once you have overcome your initial inhibitions, you will see that it is incredibly liberating – and will intensify your pleasure.

Maybe you also have a few ideas of your own, or talk to a friend for inspiration. Be open to experiments.

Sex is something each couple has to learn for themselves. Whether they suffer from vaginismus or not. Every couple develops their own "language of love", their own form or sexuality. Every couple needs to battle their way through times that are less enjoyable. The art of a fulfilling sex life consists of jointly discovering this form of "body communication" and to open up to and to stay open to new, sensual experiences.

Invest in literature

There are countless books that deal in a loving way with sexuality and sexual practices. Why not go to a bookshop and browse for a book that appeals to you? This can then provide inspiration for you and your partner to experiment.

YOUR NEXT VISIT TO THE GYNAECOLOGIST

For many women suffering from vaginismus a visit to the gynaecologist is nothing short of a nightmare. But you have reached your goal, you have beaten vaginismus. This means that you are now also capable of undergoing a gynaecological examination, pain-free.

To stay healthy, it is very important for a woman to regularly undergo a gynaecological examination. The annual check-up is a precautionary measure and ensures proper treatment of many gynaecological disorders such as inflammations, fungal infections and cysts, but also of breast cancer or cervical cancer. Of course you can also ask your gynaecologist any questions you might have about contraception, maternity and much more.

What happens during a gynaecological examination?

- **During the annual check-up,** your gynaecologist will examine your cervix, your vagina and your uterus to make sure there are no changes or disorders. Your gynaecologist will also examine your breasts and possibly your ovaries.

- **During the so-called "Pap test"** or "smear test" you usually sit in the special gynaecologist's chair. The doctor inserts a speculum into your vagina, opens it slightly and fixes it. This way your cervix becomes visible. She will then insert a little stick that is slightly rough at the end and scrape off a little mucous from your cervix. This cervical smear is then sent off to a laboratory to be examined.

- **The gynaecologist will either examine** your uterus using ultrasound or with her hands. For the ultrasound an ultrasound transducer is inserted and moved back and forth a little. This way she can see your Fallopian tubes and ovaries. With the help of ultrasound she can also locate possible cysts, myomas or similar mutations. If your gynaecologist has no ultrasound unit, she can also insert a finger into your vagina and palpate your stomach to examine your uterus.

- **Finally, your gynaecologist will palpate** your breasts and armpits. This is your breast cancer screening. She may also examine your urine or your blood.

I have compiled a few tips for your next visit to a gynaecologist. These have helped many other women to overcome their fear of the examination:

Before your first appointment

- Speak to friends, your mother, your sister. Ask which doctor they go to and what kind of experiences they have had.

- When you have chosen a doctor and are making an appointment, point out that you need time for the examination, ideally 30 minutes.

- Write down the things that are important to you. Do you want your doctor to listen to you? Do you have questions you would like to ask your doctor? Do you want your doctor to carefully explain every step? Do you want to hold the speculum (the device for the gynaecological examination) in your hands first and have it explained? Do you want to insert the speculum yourself? Many gynaecologists will respect your wish and let you insert the speculum yourself. Do you want to try sitting on the gynaecologist's chair with your clothes on first?

- Take this piece of paper along to your appointment to make sure you won't forget anything in all the excitement.

- And, to boost your confidence: practise with the dilators directly before your appointment.

- At the gynaecologist's surgery

- By all means, explain to your gynaecologist why and of what you are afraid.

- Tell her that you have suffered from vaginismus and that you have beaten the condition with the help of this book. Only if you inform your doctor about this will she know that she needs to be especially gentle and careful during the gynaecological examination. Or that she needs to choose a smaller speculum right from the start.

- Ask your doctor to explain the examination to you carefully. Ask her to announce every step of the gynaecological examination before actually performing them.

- When your doctor inserts the speculum: remember the relaxation exercises. Concentrate on your breathing. Breathe in and out calmly. Relax your pelvic floor. Relax your stomach, your bottom, your shoulders, your face.

After the appointment

You have successfully come out of your visit to the gynaecologist? You feel good and invigorated from jumping this final hurdle so easily? Then celebrate this feeling and this success! Treat yourself to something extra special – you have beaten vaginismus.

I now wish you lots of courage and all the best for your next gynaecological examination!

Regular appointments with your gynaecologist

In the past, were your examinations very painful or were vaginal examinations even impossible? Are you still afraid of gynaecological examinations? Make several appointments at three- to four-month intervals until your fear subsides somewhat and you can undergo vaginal examinations without much difficulty.

Note: In this book, I always talk of the gynaecologist as a female doctor. This is only due to the fact that the majority of women who suffer from or have suffered from vaginismus go to a female gynaecologist. This by no means implies that a male gynaecologist cannot or should not be your doctor.

PART 3:
FREQUENTLY ASKED
QUESTIONS

Every week I receive emails from women who suffer from vaginismus or from their partners. Some questions are very personal and some women elaborate in detail on their own "vaginismus history". Other questions come up frequently, but still cause uncertainty in many women or couples.

Contents

116

Q: I would like to present and clarify the most common questions here. You will find answers on the following pages.

During psychotherapy I was introduced to autogenic training. Can I also practise this instead of PMR?

A: If you are still familiar with the exercises, you can of course also use autogenic training to relax. However, give progressive muscle relaxation a try, too. This technique works with the different muscle groups that are often also tensed up or cause cramps.

Q: I'm not really relaxed after practising PMR. On the contrary, sometimes I feel even more tensed up. Am I doing something wrong?

A: You are probably building up too strong a tension. Bring the respective body parts into the described starting position first. Without force, without tension, almost imperceptibly. Wait for two to three breaths and observe where in your body you can feel tension. Slowly and veeery, very gently build up a mini-tension. Wait again for two to three breaths and once again observe where in your body you can feel tension or even tensed up areas. Very slowly and carefully release the tension when you next breathe out: for example, let your shoulder sink back into its starting position.

Q: A therapist recommended osteopathy to me as a treatment for vaginismus. I started a week ago, and I really feel more relaxed now. Can I skip the vaginal training now?

A: Whether or not you practise osteopathy, acupuncture, shiatsu, connective tissue massage, yoga, qigong or the Feldenkrais Method, a vaginal and pelvic floor training is sadly inevitable if you want to successfully beat vaginismus. Nevertheless, the above mentioned methods are really great to support you during your vaginismus therapy, as a stress management measure, to relax, to keep your inner balance or to strengthen your mental wellbeing.

Q: I am not sure I am tensing my pelvic floor properly.

A: Stay with the juggling ball exercise for a bit longer. Keep reaching for your sitting bones and check whether you can feel a slightly increased tension between your sitting bones. In addition, use the hand mirror and pulsate with your pelvic floor muscles. You are really working with your whole pelvic floor, when you can see your perineum arching gently (!) inwards and when the area between your sitting bones contracts a little.

For more pelvic floor exercise tips, please see the workbook and accompanying diary "Wenn die Liebe schmerzt" [When love hurts].

Q: I am afraid to make mistakes when doing the pelvic floor exercises and to worsen my condition. Can I simply enrol for a pelvic floor exercise class at the adult education centre?

A: Sadly only very few instructors are familiar with the topic of vaginismus. Traditional pelvic floor training teaches – as described earlier – the typical tube feeling and mainly exercises the outer and middle muscle layer of the pelvic floor. Instructors who are familiar with vaginismus and vulvodynia can be found at www.genito-pelvic-pain.com.

Q: The vaginal training with the dilators is very painful or I get this burning sensation, so I don't really want to practise anymore.

A: Go back to the beginning again. Focus on the pelvic floor training and the relaxation exercises. Can you feel your pelvic floor easily? Can you cope alright with the exercises? Choose just one exercise, but do it precisely, well and in a relaxed way. Only start with the dilator training again, when you can insert your finger without feeling any pain.

Q: I always get this slight burning sensation when I do the vaginal training, even after I have finished practising. I suspect the lubricant – is that possible?

A: A burning sensation is usually a sign of strongly tensed pelvic floor muscles. Often, women do not perceive this tension in their pelvic floor and, when training with the dilators, they feel as if their vaginal mucous membrane were burning. Once the tension in the pelvic floor becomes less – also during the vaginal training – the burning sensation will subside completely. Take note of the tension in your pelvic floor as often as possible. At work, while chatting to a friend, while watching TV, while queuing at the checkout. What is the tension like in your pelvic floor? Tense or medium tense or relaxed? If you would like to try a different lubricant all the same, the perfume- and additive-free water- or silicone-based lubricants are ideal.

Q: I suffer from vulvodynia and am experiencing severe pain during the vaginal training. Should I practise with the dilators nonetheless?

A: Yes and no. Train your pelvic floor as often as possible – as always with minimum strength. Integrate the training into your day-to-day life: for example, pulsate 30 to 40 times when you sit down or after you have gone to the toilet, every morning in bed or when you are watching a film ...

Do not practise with the dilators for too long. Sometimes five minutes (ideally daily) are enough to be able to practise without pain. Reread the chapter on "Hints for using the self-help programme against vulvodynia" and apply them.

Q: I have finally beaten vaginismus with the help of this book. I can have sex now, but I cannot enjoy it yet.

A: If you have only completed the programme a short while ago, give yourself and your body a little time to accept and process the new sensations and feelings. Talk openly to your partner about your emotions. It is most helpful to throw any sense of shame overboard and to start masturbating. Take plenty of time and keep your body completely relaxed. This way you will learn which forms of contact arouse you, and you can pass these discoveries on to your partner.

Often couples take sexual intercourse much too seriously once they have beaten vaginismus together. But there is no such thing as "correct sex". Of course it will help you to overcome fears if you practise sex as often as possible. But sexuality should and may, above all, be pleasurable. Indulge in other sexual practices, too, and do not fixate exclusively on sexual intercourse. Not every sexual encounter needs to be about the man's penis penetrating the woman's vagina.

Explore one another's preferences and find out what arouses you sexually. The more aroused you are before "inserting the penis", the easier it will be for you to enjoy sex.

If you have already completed the programme a while ago and nothing has changed since, do not hesitate to ask for advice from a sex therapist.

Q: The largest dilator in the Amielle Set is a little smaller than my partner's erect penis. I have no problem inserting the largest dilator and feel no pain, but it simply won't work with my partner. Are there any larger dilators I could buy?

A: Yes, there are. But the size of the largest dilator is usually enough, even if your partner's penis is a little bigger. Try repeating every step of the PMR, the pelvic floor exercises and the final partner exercises again. How about sub-dividing the steps of the exercises into even smaller steps? Practise with the dilators again directly before the partner exercises so that your pelvic floor is well and truly relaxed. Many women also find a different position helpful for inserting the penis. If you really feel that the largest dilator is too small, you can find contact details on our homepage for a dealer who sells larger dilators. You can, of course, also simply order a dildo or vibrator you like and practise with a new size this way.

Q: I have read about the trigger point therapy on the internet. What is this?

A: In physiotherapy, "trigger points" are described as tiny areas in the muscles that trigger pain. Such pressure points often develop through chronic tension, over-strained muscles or through stress. Pressing such a point usually triggers a severe, stabbing pain that subsides again after a while. The pressure reduces the blood circulation for a moment, however, circulation is immediately resumed once you let go. This relaxes the muscle and, after a while, produces a soothing effect. Trigger points can be located directly around the painful area, but also far away from it.

If you are not too pain-sensitive, you can detect such trigger points in your lower back, your groin, around the perineum or even inside your vagina by systematically pressing down on your tissue inch by inch. The trigger point therapy consists of pressing on the painful spots until the pain subsides. The area may subsequently continue to feel pressure-sensitive and painful. The trigger point therapy can be a good way to support the vaginismus therapy. However, it cannot beat vaginismus on its own.

Q: We would like to have a baby. What should I bear in mind during the pregnancy and birth?

A: In principle, there are no special pregnancy rules for women who have success-fully beaten vaginismus. But, by all means, go to antenatal classes with your partner so that you are well prepared for the birth. Also tell your gynaecologist and midwife that you suffered from vaginismus in the past.

YOUR NEXT STEPS

Learn what it takes to overcome sexual pain

This book is about how to overcome successful vaginismus, vulvodynia, sexual pain after surgery or after giving birth. Learning what it takes to succeed helps to stay tuned to the self-treatment and to combat fears of treatment failure.

Do the exercises

Take action. Do the steps you've learned. It's one thing to read and to know and quite another to put what you know into action. Taking action is the only way to overcome sexual pain and fear of penetration. That's why it's so important to follow the steps and just do the exercises.

Beware of that little voice in your head that says things like "I can't do it" and "I have no time" or "it's too hard".

Yes it takes time, practice and effort. But if you are willing to follow these 7 simple Steps and don't give up when you run into challenges or setbacks - you will be amazed by the results, just like so many women who've followed this programme have been.

Share

The best way to keep on track and make this programme a part of your everyday life is to share your success with your family, your loved ones and with your friends.

Commit to tell about this programme your doctor, physical therapist, sexual therapist, psychotherapist and other healthcare specialists whom you sought for help.

Commit to share with women affected by sexual pain or chronic pelvic pain to help them overcoming these conditions. Encourage them to purchase copies so they can begin their own life-changing journey to beat penetration disorders, vaginismus and other chronic pelvic pain conditions.

Share your experiences with me to help improve the programme. And I love to hear success stories! No matter where you are, share your story at www.genito-pelvic-pain.com or at our facebook fanpage or in the private facebook-group "vaginismus besiegen".

PART **4:**
INFORMATION FOR
PRACTITIONERS

Contents

THE PELVIC FLOOR

The images of the pelvic floor in the second part of the book are labelled, where possible, with common names. In the interests of clarity, you will find these images reproduced again on the following pages, but this time with the Latin muscle names.

Diagnosis criteria for vaginismus and dyspareunia

The DSM-IV-TR is currently being revised, and the new edition should come out in 2012/2013 as DSM-5. In the course of this revision, the diagnosis criteria and categorisation for vaginismus and dyspareunia have been under debate. A renewal of the approach to vaginismus, dyspareunia and vulvodynia is long overdue: the current diagnosis criteria in the ICD-10 and DSM-IV are outdated and have been proven partly or completely wrong in a number of studies. The proposed guidelines are clearer, more differentiated and more practical. Consequently, the diagnosis and therapy would de facto be easier to implement for doctors and therapists than with the existing criteria.

My work, the therapy programme 'Vaginismus besiegen®' [beat vaginismus] and the therapists trained by me all follow the newly proposed guidelines. I would therefore like to give you an overview here.

Images of the pelvic floor with Latin names for the muscles

Traditionally, the pelvic floor is divided into the Diaphragma urogenitale and the Diaphragma pelvis. We follow newer descriptions and differentiate between three muscle layers of the pelvic floor:

- the outer layer, the muscles of which cover the erectile tissue of the clitoris and anus,

- the perineal membrane or middle layer,

- the levator ani or inner layer.

Subdividing the pelvic floor into three layers makes especially great sense when considering the research results on the anatomy of the clitoris by the urologist and surgeon Dr. Helen O'Connell[2].

In the following, you will find images of the three layers of the pelvic floor again, but this time with the Latin muscle names.

---

[2] Helen E. O'Connell, John M. Hutson, Colin R. Anderson and Robert J. Plenter, Anatomical relationship between urethra and clitoris, Journal of Urology, Vol. 159, June 1998.

PELVIC FLOOR: OUTER LAYER

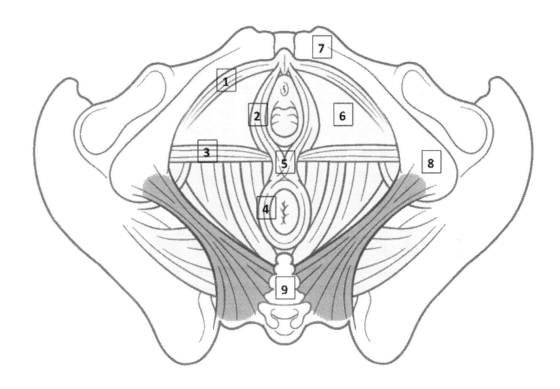

1 M. ischiocavernosus (ischiocavernosus muscle)

2 M. bulbospongiosus (bulbospongiosus muscle)

3 M. transversus perinei superficialis (superficial transverse perineal muscle)

4 M. sphincter ani externus (external anal sphincter)

5 Centrum perinei (perineum)

6 Perineal membrane (middle layer)

7 Symphysis pubica (pubic bone)

8 Tuber ischiadicum (Tuberosity of the ischium or sitting bones)

9 Os coccygis (coccyx)

➟ see also step 2:
The outer or lower layer 37

PELVIC FLOOR: MIDDLE LAYER

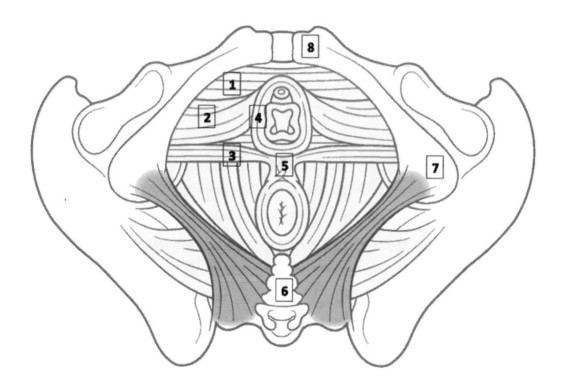

1 M. transversus perinei profundus
(deep transverse perineal muscle)

2 M. compressor urethrae (urethral
sphincter)

3 M. transversus perinei superficialis
(superficial transverse perineal
muscle), outer layer

4 M. sphincter urethrovaginalis
(urethrovaginal sphincter)

5 Centrum perinei (perineum)

6 Os coccygis (coccyx)

7 Tuber ischiadicum (Tuberosity of the
ischium or sitting bones)

8 Symphysis pubica (pubic bone)

⇒ see also step 2:
The middle layer page #38

PELVIC FLOOR: INNER LAYER

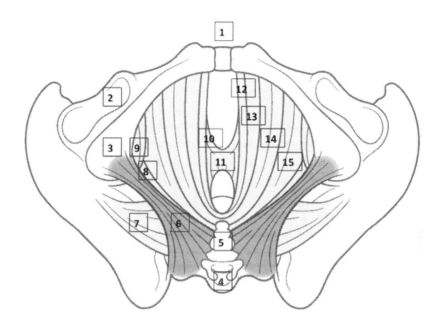

1 Symphysis pubica (pubic bone)

2 hip joint

3 Tuber ischiadicum (Tuberosity of the ischium or sitting bones)

4 os sacrum (sacral bone)

5 Os coccygis (coccyx)

6 Lig. sacrotuberale (great or posterior sacrosciatic ligament)

7 M. piriformis ("pear shaped" muscle)

8 M. ischiococcygeus (ischiococcygeus muscle, sitting bone-to-coccyx muscle)

9 M. obturator internus (obturator internus muscle)

10 M. pubovaginalis – part of the levator ani (pubovaginalis muscle, pubic-bone-to-vagina muscle)

11 M. puboperinealis (puboperinealis muscle, pubic-bone-to-perineum muscle)

12 M. puboanalis – part of the levator ani (pubovaginalis muscle, pubic-bone-to-anus muscle)

13 M. puborectalis – part of the levator ani (puborectalis or sphincter recti)

14 M. pubococcygeus – part of the levator ani (pubococcygeus or PC muscle, pubic-bone-to-coccyx muscle)

15 M. iliococcygeus – part of the levator ani (iliococcygeus muscle, ilium-to-coccyx muscle)

➡ see also step 2:
The inner layer page # 39

THE PELVIC ORGANS

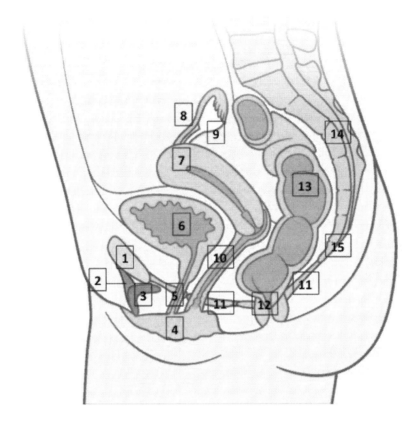

1 Symphysis pubica (pubic bone)

2 Ligamentum suspensorium clitoridis
(suspensory ligament of the clitoris)

3 Corpus clitoridis (part of the clitoris)

4 Labia majora pudendi (labia)

5 Urethra

6 Vesica urinaria (bladder)

7 Corpus uteri (uterus)

8 Tuba uterina (Fallopian tube)

9 Ovarium (ovary)

10 Vagina

11 Pelvic floor

12 Canalis analis (anus)

13 Intestinum (rectum) (intestine)

14 Os sacrum (sacral bone)

15 Os coccygis (coccyx)

⇒ see also step 4:
A little anatomy page #63

THE CLITORIS

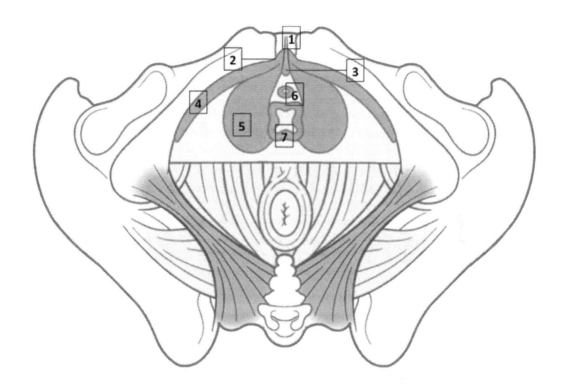

1 Ligamentum suspensorium clitoridis (suspensory ligament of the clitoris)

2 Corpus clitoridis (clitoral body)

3 Glans clitoridis (clitoral glans)

Crus clitoridis (clitoral crura) - part of the corpus cavernosum clitoridis which is attached to the perineal membrane

4 Corpus cavernosum clitoridis (clitoral crura)

5 Bulbus vestibuli (clitoral bulb)

6 Clitoral tissue surrounding the urethra

8 Clitoral tissue surrounding the vagina

9 Glandula paraurethralis (Skene's gland)

10 Glandula vestibularis major (Bartholin gland)

⟹ see also step 4: Clitoris page #64

CORONAL PLANE OF THE PELVIS

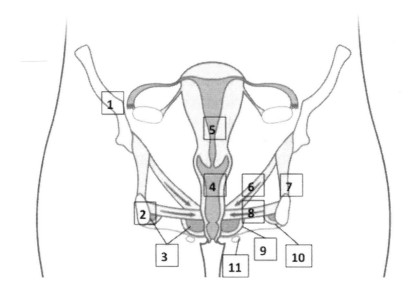

1 Os ilium (ilium bone)

2 Tuber ischiadicum (Tuberosity of the ischium or sitting bone)

3 Bulbus vestibuli (clitoral bulb)

4 Vagina

5 Corpus unteri (uterus)

6 Levator ani (levator ani muscles)

7 M. obturator internus (obturator internus muscle)

8 Perineal membrane (middle layer)

9 M. bulbospongiosus (bulbospongio-sus muscle)

10 M. ischiocavernosus (ischiocaverno-sus muscle)

➡ see also step 4: page #65

VAGINISMUS AND DYSPAREUNIA: SEXUAL OR PAIN DISORDER?

Usually, ailments are categorised according to their symptoms and not according to the activity during which they occur, as is the case with vaginismus and dyspareunia. For example, stomach ache would never be classed as a sexual disorder, even if stomach ache is regularly triggered during sexual intercourse. A similar situation: pain in connection with vaginismus and dyspareunia. Often, the pain not only occurs during sexual intercourse, but also in other situations that involve vaginal penetration, e.g. a vaginal gynaecological examination, when inserting a tampon or even when the woman tries to insert her own finger. Consequently, the question of whether vaginismus and dyspareunia should in fact be classed as pain disorders is justifiable.

Vaginismus

For more than 150 years, the diagnosis criterion for vaginismus has been spasms in the muscles of the outer third of the vagina or spasms in part of the pelvic floor muscles. In the three studies that have to date been published on this topic, spasms of the pelvic floor muscles could not be detected in all women suffering from vaginismus. Spasms of the pelvic floor muscles were not much more common in women with vaginismus than in the group of women without vaginismus.

However, practically all women suffering from vaginismus displayed an increased muscle tone. If spasms of the pelvic floor cease to count as diagnosis criteria for vaginismus, naturally the question arises, which criteria should apply and whether a distinction between vaginismus and dyspareunia should be made at all.

Dyspareunia

In recent years, dyspareunia was often divided into superficial dyspareunia and deep dyspareunia. Superficial dyspareunia being the broader term for disorders such as vulvodynia or vulvar vestibulitis; deep dyspareunia being the broader term for disorders such as endometriosis, levator ani syndrome or interstitial cystitis.

Symptoms frequently overlap, which is why no clear diagnosis can be given based on the symptoms.

Genito-pelvic pain/penetration disorder

The current hodge-podge of diagnoses and the communication mayhem between doctors, therapists and patients could be simplified by summarising the disorders under the umbrella term of genito-pelvic pain/penetration disorder. According to Binik[4], the new diagnosis criteria in the DSM-5 could read as follows:

A Persistent or recurrent difficulties for at least 6 months with one or more of the following:

1) Inability to have vaginal intercourse/penetration on at least 50 percent of attempts.

2) Marked genito-pelvic pain during at least 50 percent of vaginal intercourse/penetration attempts.

3) Marked fear of vaginal intercourse/penetration or of genito-pelvic pain during intercourse/penetration on at least 50% of vaginal intercourse/penetration attempts.

4) Marked tensing or tightening of the pelvic floor muscles during attempted vaginal intercourse/penetration on at least 50 percent of occasions.

B The disorder causes significant psychological strain or interpersonal problems.

Defining diagnosis A and B in more detail

General medical disorder, e.g. Lichen sclerosus or endometriosis.

With years of experience as an expert in treating women with genito-pelvic pain, I can attest that their descriptions of their symptoms frequently cannot be clearly attributed to vaginismus, dyspareunia or vulvodynia. Not least because of this, many women spend years searching for a diagnosis and a suitable therapy to treat their disorder. Summarising these disorders under the term of genito-pelvic pain/penetration disorder will make it easier for doctors to make a diagnosis and for therapists to compile a suitable therapy. In addition, the above approach clearly shows when additional cooperation from doctors is necessary.

In future, the following description will probably replace the current diagnosis guidelines for vaginismus and dyspareunia in the DSM-IV (the release of DSM-5 will be in mai 2013):

---

[4] Yitzchak M. Binik, The DSM Diagnostic Criteria for Dyspareunia, Springer 2009; The DSM Diagnostic Criteria for Vaginismus, Springer 2009.

DSM-V: GENITO-PELVIC PAIN/PENETRATION DISORDER

A. Persistent or recurrent difficulties for at least 6 months with one or more of the following:

1) Marked difficulty having vaginal intercourse/penetration

2) Marked vulvovaginal or pelvic pain during vaginal intercourse/penetration attempts

3) Marked fear or anxiety either about vulvovaginal or pelvic pain or vaginal penetration

4) Marked tensing or tightening of the pelvic floor muscles during attempted vaginal penetration

A. The problem causes clinically significant distress or impairment

B. The sexual dysfunction is not attributable to a non-sexual psychiatric disorder, by the effects of a substance/medication, by another medical condition, by severe relationship distress (e.g., partner violence), or other significant stressors.

Subtype: Lifelong vs. acquired

Specifiers:

1) Generalized vs. situational

2) With concomitant problems in sexual interest/sexual arousal

3) Partner factors (partner's sexual problems, partner's health status)

4) Relationship factors (e.g., poor communication, discrepancies in desire for sexual activity)

5) Individual vulnerability factors or psychiatric co-morbidity (e.g., depression or anxiety, poor body image, history of abuse experience)

6) Cultural/religious factors (e.g., inhibitions related to prohibitions against sexual activity)

7) With medical factors relevant to prognosis, course, or treatment

The revised diagnosis guidelines in the DSM-5 (Diagnostic and Statistical Manual of Mental Disorders) are clearer and more precise than the present classifications in the ICD-10/DSM-IV for vaginismus and dyspareunia.

In practice, the symptoms of vaginismus and dyspareunia are often almost indistinguishable. For this reason, many women seeking help spend years trying to get a diagnosis, let alone a suitable treatment.

We work according to the guidelines set for genito-pelvic pain in the DSM-5 and recommend doctors, if asked to give a diagnosis based on the respective symptoms, to also follow the DSM-5 and to only diagnose dyspareunia and, in particular, vaginismus if absolutely necessary.

Proposal

The existing data suggest a lack of reliability for the current DSM-IV-TR diagnoses of Vaginismus and Dyspareunia and the inability to differentially diagnose these two disorders. The current proposed category is descriptive and intended to reflect this situation and provide a framework to facilitate clinician diagnosis and assessment as well as to allow for the inclusion of women suffering from pain and penetration difficulties into the DSM-5.

DSM-IV

Genito-Pelvic Pain/Penetration Disorder includes previous diagnoses of Vaginismus (Not Due to a General Medical Condition) and Dyspareunia (Not Due to a General Medical Condition).

CONTACT THE AUTHOR

Claudia Amherd

www.moyosecrets.info

REFERENCES

Yitzchak M. Binik. The DSM Diagnostic Criteria for Dyspareunia; Springer 2009. The DSM Diagnostic Criteria for Vaginismus; Springer 2009

Dyspareunia Looks Sexy on First But How Much Pain Will It Take for It to Score? A Reply to My Critics Concerning the DSM Classification of Dyspareunia as a Sexual Dysfunction. Archives of Sexual Behavior, Volume 34, Number 1, February 2005, 63–67

Should Dyspareunia Be Retained as a Sexual Dysfunction in DSM-V? A Painful Classification Decision. Archives of Sexual Behavior, Volume 34, Number 1, February 2005, 11–21

Kimberley A. Payne, Sophie Bergeron, Samir Khalifé, Yitzchak M. Binik. Assessment, Treatment Strategies, and Outcome Results: Perspective of Pain Specialist. 12-Goldstein-chs12-ppp, August 2005, 473–481

Physical Therapy for Vulvar Vestibulitis Syndrome: A Retrospective Study. Journal of Sex & Marital Therapy, 2002, 28: 183–192

Alessandra Graziottin. Sexual Pain Disorders: Dyspareunia and Vaginismus in: Porst H. Buvat J. (Eds), ISSM (International Society of Sexual Medicine)Standard Committee Book, Standard Practice in Sexual Medicine, Blackwell, Oxford, UK, 2006, 342–350

Gayle Watts, and Daniel Nettle. The Role of Anxiety in Vaginismus: A Case-Control Study Newcastle University, Institute of Neuroscience, Newcastle, United Kingdom, June 2009, 1–6

Tessa Crowley, David Goldmeier, Janice Hiller. Diagnosing and Managing Vaginismus-British Medical Journal, June 2009

M. Mousavi Nasab, Z. Farnoosh- Management of Vaginismus with Cognitive –Behavioral Therapy, Self-Finger Approach: A Study of 70 Cases- Iranian Journal of Medical Sciences, Volume 28, June 2003, Number 2, 69–71

T. Y. Rosenbaum- The Role of Physiotherapy in Sexual Health: Is it Evidence-Based? Urogynecological Physiotherapy, Tel Aviv and Jerusalem, Israel, Journal of the Association of Chartered Physiotherapists in Women's Health, Autumn 2006, 1–5

Musculoskeletal Pain and Sexual Function in Women. Inner Stability, Urogynecological Physiotherapy, Bet Shemesh, Israel, 2009, 1–6

Pelvic Floor Involvement in Male and Female Sexual Dysfunctionand the Role of Pelvic Floor Rehabilitation in Treatment: A Literature Review. Urogynecological Physiotherapy Private Practice, Tel Aviv and Jerusalem, Israel, Journal of Sex Medicine, 2007, 4: 4–13

Rosenbaum T. Y., and Owens. AThe Role of Pelvic Floor Physical Therapy in the Treatment of Pelvic and Genital Pain-Related Sexual Dysfunction. Journal of Sex Medicine, 2008, 5: 513–523

Kimberly A. Fisher. Management of Dyspareunia and Associated Levator Ani Muscle

Overactivity; Physical Therapy, 2007, 87: 935–941

E. Lambreva, R. Klaghofer, C. Buddeberg. Psychosoziale Aspekte bei Patientinnen und Patienten mit sexuellen FunktionsstörungenPraxis, 2006, 95: 226–231

Made in the USA
Middletown, DE
31 March 2018